Anders [...] nish–Irish parentage. He [...] ear[ly] years trav[elling, then got] stuck in the hab[it] and [...] car[...]in. [He has] taught English in Abu Dhabi and Mexico, played volleyball for Ireland, and has had jobs ranging from lavatory cleaner in New York to demolition worker in Munich. But he is not – nor has ever been – a barber. He currently lives in Ireland with his family, where he practises karate and wishes it didn't rain so much.

Sharp Practice

THE REAL MAN'S GUIDE TO SHAVING

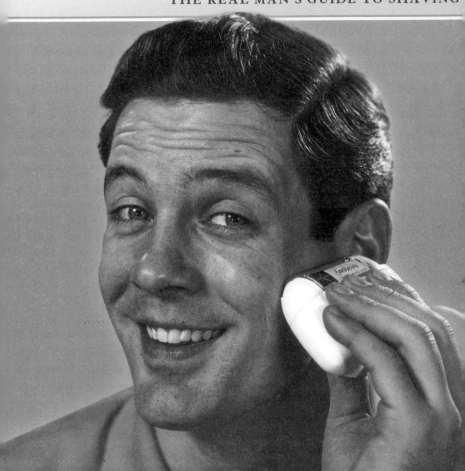

ANDERS LARSEN

CORGI BOOKS

TRANSWORLD PUBLISHERS
61–63 Uxbridge Road, London W5 5SA
a division of The Random House Group Ltd
www.booksattransworld.co.uk

SHARP PRACTICE
A CORGI BOOK: 9780552155076

First published in Great Britain
in 2006 by Bantam Press
a division of Transworld Publishers
Corgi edition published 2007

A CIP catalogue record for this book
is available from the British Library

Addresses for Random House Group Ltd companies outside the UK
can be found at: www.randomhouse.co.uk
The Random House Group Ltd Reg. No. 954009

The Random House Group Ltd makes every effort to ensure that the papers used in its
books are made from trees that have been legally sourced from well-managed and
credibly certified forests. Our paper procurement policy can be found at:
www.randomhouse.co.uk/paper.htm

Book designed and illustrated by Lynnette Eve
www.design-jam.co.uk

Typeset in 11/15pt Egyptian 505 by
Falcon Oast Graphic Art Ltd.

Printed in the UK by CPI Bookmarque, Croydon, CR0 4TD

2 4 6 8 10 9 7 5 3 1

To Trisha,
who hasn't turfed out this old rapscallion yet

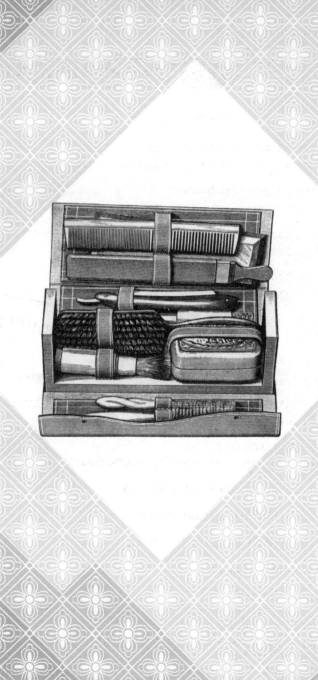

CONTENTS

Sharp Practice

THE REAL MAN'S GUIDE TO SHAVING

> 'To shave the beard is a sin that the blood
> of all the martyrs cannot cleanse.'
>
> **Ivan the Terrible, Tsar of Russia**

Shaving?

I started when I was about sixteen. A school disco was coming up, and I thought I had a chance with a girl I knew. I looked in the mirror and decided it was time to take off that fluff – time to become a man.

I didn't own an electric, so I went down to the supermarket and picked up a cheap disposable razor and a can of shaving foam. It didn't cost much.

Nobody offered advice, then or at any time in the future. Apart from anything else, I never asked. Instinctively, I knew that real men had to go through this on their own. Like St George off to fight my dragon, I entered the bathroom – my battlefield – certain that I would emerge victorious. I was going to look like Marlon Brando, Robert Redford, maybe even John Wayne. That girl was as good as mine.

Half an hour later I was rinsing bloodstains off the washbasin, and my face looked like I'd stuck it in a blender. And after I'd finished with the blade? Here came the good part: I could splash on the aftershave, and the sweet scent would compensate for everything. It would make me smell like a man at least.

Splash, splash.

'AAARGH!'

Napalm.

When the raw alcohol burned into my face, my knees buckled and, to my eternal shame, I wept. The pain was appalling. I had no idea that this was what it took to be a man. Why didn't women have to do it?

Oh, and I blamed my razor for the fact that my girl went off with some gorilla awash with testosterone who'd been shaving since he was twelve.

If this type of beginning sounds chaotic, be advised that it's also the standard first shave for most men.

And the bizarre thing is this: we don't ask for advice on shaving *ever*. We go through years of learning the hard way. We turn thirty, but still don't ask our best friend what type of razor, shaving brush, soap or aftershave he uses. It's taboo. We walk around the streets with nicks, cuts, razor-burn and the stubbly bits we missed or skipped in sensitive areas. To advertise them, we stick on bits of lavatory paper to flap in the breeze like little red and white flags.

And that, my friend, is the tragic story of nearly the entire male population of the Western world. They've never been taught and, God help them, half don't have a clue.

*

This book will tell you how to shave, whether with an electric, a safety or a cut-throat.

Oh, you've been shaving for years, and you know all this?

Then you know all about honing, stropping, lathering and silver-tip badger? And you know about alum, styptic, linen, horsehide and Russian reds, monoterpenes and the stratum corneum, second and third passes, high carbon and stainless steel? How about Japanese Waterstone, Belgian Blackstone or Norton, 4000/8000 grit, madder root, aftershave lotions v. balms, King Camp Gillette, Colonel Conk and Dominica Bay Rum?

No, I didn't think so.

But let's face it: a book that was only about shaving would be hellish boring. So I've put in bits about Alexander the Great tossing severed heads about, Che Guevara smoking cigars in the jungle with Fidel Castro, and how I was attacked in an opium den by a Chinese man with a machete.

Confused? You will be. Read on.

The way I see it, there are three different ways of shaving:

- the electric razor
- the safety razor
- the cut-throat razor.

I'll go through them all, but I'll start with the cut-throat since I use one myself and have done for years. (No, it's not dangerous at all.)

Here's how that happened.

THE OLD CURIOSITY SHOP

It was a different age.

November rain sleeted across my face, through my hair and down my upturned collar. I was running for shelter – an overhang on the far side of the street – my feet splashing through monster puddles, my cheap shoes soaked.

Safe from the rain, I patted down my pockets and fished out a dry cigarette. A sign in a window caught my eye: The Oldest Shop in Dublin. Strange: after eight years I'd thought I knew Dublin quite well, yet I'd never noticed that sign before. It looked like a shabby old men's shop, and I was intrigued. I pushed open the door and walked in, cigarette dangling from my lips.

That shop has long since closed down, but I still remember some of the details clearly. The display cases were dark wood, mahogany or teak, and well oiled. The floor was glossy tiles, black and white squares. The glass cases were full of steel and leather: hunting knives, carving knives and penknives. They had some switchblades on display. There may have been a sword or two. There were leather cases, hip flasks, hand-stitched boots and walking-sticks. A no-frills men's shop.

No one else was in there. I wandered down to the far end of the counter, not intending to buy anything. I remember wiping my face dry on my sleeve and having another pull on my cigarette. Back then we smoked in shops.

That was when it stopped me: a dull light fell on it, catching my eye. I was transfixed.

The shopkeeper shuffled over. He had white hair and a wrinkled face, and a pipe hung out of his mouth. 'It's what separates the men from the boys, sonny.'

We eyed each other through the drifting smoke.

'The disposables they sell now,' he muttered. 'They're for disposable men.'

'How much?'

I can't remember the price he told me. I was always terrible with money and still am. But it certainly wasn't more than ten pounds. That doesn't seem like a lot now, but I was a student then, and poor.

I rooted out the money in coins and notes, and the old man wrapped the blade in brown paper. There was no case, but it came with a strop, the essential strip of leather that keeps the blade dry and correctly aligned. It served me well, and the shopkeeper gave me advice: 'Always strop after you finish the shave, sonny. It's German, high-carbon steel. You don't have to worry about sharpening it. They stay sharp for years.'

It was male advice: short, to the point, transactional. We didn't need to chatter.

I dropped the blade into my pocket and ambled back to the door. When I had it half open, he called after me: 'Brando!'

I turned round. The old man was grinning. 'Marlon Brando used one. *Last Tango in Paris*. It's a great movie.'

I grinned back. 'I've seen it.'

Once outside, I flicked my cigarette butt into the gutter and turned my collar down again. The rain had stopped. Sunlight was fighting its way through the clouds. My hand brushed against the razor in my pocket. It felt like a friend.

*

I've used that razor for a long time now. It's travelled with me through Mexico, the Persian Gulf and the jungles of Thailand. It's been through wars and ditches. I was forty metres under water once when I realized I had forgotten to take it out of my pocket before diving at an oil-rig.

I've tried other blades, of course, but that one always draws me back. I think, at this point, there won't be another.

'And so,' you ask, 'where can I purchase one?'

Easy: you can lay your hands on a cut-throat razor in several different ways:

- You can find one in an old shop, like I did. This is a lot of fun, and it's a great way to buy one, as long as you take on board a few warnings, as you'll see below.

- You can buy one on the Internet. This might be the easiest option, if you feel comfortable buying things on the Internet.

- You can buy one in an old flea market. Be warned: this is a dangerous option and you should select it only if you know what you're doing.

TOBY'S GRIZZLY BEAR

I had a stockbroker friend, Toby, who really liked the idea of the cut-throat razor. I was in London for the summer and we were having a few drinks together. In fact, we drank a lot. The lights grew dimmer and we approached that magical time of night when every word makes sense. I told Toby how it all worked – what to do and what to avoid – and I could see a crazy gleam in his eye at the very idea of the cut-throat razor. Looking back, of course, I should have warned him, as I'm warning you now.

That same weekend, Toby had arranged for us to go to a stockbroker's dinner-dance. I'd rented a tux, finished a fantastic shave and celebrated by splashing Colonel Conk aftershave all over my face.

Toby called me up as I was struggling into my tux. 'I can't make it.'

'What?'

'Something's come up. You'll have to go alone.'

This was going to be a disaster. I knew there was no chance I'd have a good night without him. I didn't know any other stockbrokers, and I was nearly certain I didn't have anything in common with them. My after-dinner conversation is about things normal people find barely acceptable.

'Dammit. What happened?'

He wouldn't say. He was humming and hawing and I was beginning to think he'd arranged something else on the sly.

This required drastic action, so I went to his apartment, which was round the corner, and I kept my finger on the buzzer until he came down.

When he opened the door, one side of his face looked as if a grizzly bear had tried to eat it. He was nearly in tears. 'I can't believe you shave with one of those horrible things.'

'Let me see the razor.'

When he showed it to me, I saw that he had gone into an antiques shop and bought an incredibly expensive one whose handle was studded with diamonds. It looked as if it had been made for the King of Sweden. But when I felt the blade, it was barely sharper than that of a kitchen knife. There was a nick in it and the edge was misaligned – a great-looking razor for a display cabinet. It was my first real experience of style over substance.

Be warned: 99 per cent of used razors need serious reconditioning work before they're going to be of any use. That's fine, if you're an expert with a hone and strop. But most people aren't. *That's why, if you're a beginner with the cut-throat razor, you should steer clear of second-hand blade*s. If you think you're going to have a positive experience using your grandfather's razor, with nicks in it and a patina of rust on the blade, think again. I'm not discrediting old blades – quite the opposite: it's rewarding to save a faithful old razor from the scrap heap and use it daily. And this can be even more important if it carries emotional weight with you. But save it until you've been using a cut-throat for years. It takes time to learn, and you'll only hurt yourself in the beginning.

Incidentally, I bought Toby a decent cut-throat a few

days later. He's been using it ever since, and now he feels as I do about the cut-throat:

- It's a beautiful, ancient instrument that is still fully functional. You could compare the experience to driving a 1920s Mercedes, but with the performance of a state-of-the-art Ferrari.
- It gives you a smoother shave than the most modern electric or safety razor.
- It reduces or eliminates razor-burn and nicks.
- It can make you feel like a craftsman – which neither a safety nor an electric razor can.
- It's a whole barrel of fun, and your wife or partner will think you're nuts.

GERMAN AND FRENCH RAZORS

So, now that you know you should buy a new razor, I have some even more specific advice: buy one made in Germany or France. This may seem cruel to other manufacturers and, indeed, other countries, but I'm basing it 100 per cent on personal experience. And I'm going to restrict your choice even further: when I say Germany, I mean 'Solingen'. This is the town in Germany where they make the best blades. If you're holding a cut-throat razor with 'Solingen' on the blade, you have a product made from some of the finest steel in the world, which has the corresponding depth of craftsmanship behind it. The name 'Solingen' has been legally protected since 1938.

The biggest Solingen brand-name is 'Dovo'. This venerable company was founded in 1906 by Herr Dorp and Herr Voos – combine the first two letters of their names and you have 'Dovo'. Over many years, 'Dovo' incorporated six other cut-throat razor manufacturers. That makes for a wealth of manufacturing experience, combined with a very high-quality product.

Dovo make cut-throat razors that will last you a lifetime. Even the cheapest of their razors will serve you well, as long as you maintain them properly. Dovo blades are also quite reasonably priced. You can investigate their models at any number of websites. From there, it's easy: you pay your money and take your pick.

So much for the German blades. When I say France, I'm being even more specific. I mean 'Thiers-Issard'. This isn't a place in France: it's a brand-name, and it stands alone. Thiers-Issard is to razors what Rolls-Royce is to cars.

This legendary company was founded by Pierre Thiers in France in about 1884. He was a barrel-chested blacksmith and spent his lifetime hammering out top-quality products at the forge, becoming a master razor-maker. He passed his knowledge and his business on to his son, also named Pierre Thiers. Various other members of the Thiers family were brought in to work in the business – it was something of a blacksmithing clan. Nowadays the company is no longer family-owned, but the quality and tradition continues unabated. They use Sheffield steel for their blades. If you want to buy a work of art, take a look at their limited editions. You won't find a better one. They're expensive, though. I suppose how much you spend depends on what type of man you are. You can investigate Thiers-Issard prices and models on the Internet too.

Now, here's the thing: I refuse to recommend any other model from any other country. I especially warn you to treat with caution razors made in certain developing countries. They may look amazing, but they're frequently made from inferior steel. And you'll feel the difference on your skin. Many are unusable.

THE FEATHER RAZOR

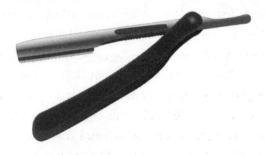

The feather razor is sometimes called a 'shavette'. It's a hybrid between a disposable and a cut-throat. It has the form of a cut-throat, but you fit a disposable blade into it. You might have seen – or felt – them used on the back of your neck in a barbershop, to clean up the tufty bits at the back of your hairline. If you feel you need that interim step, go for it.

I never did.

Having ploughed through the warnings, here's a picture of what a typical cut-throat razor should look like. I've attached the names of the parts, to make sure we're all using the same vocabulary.

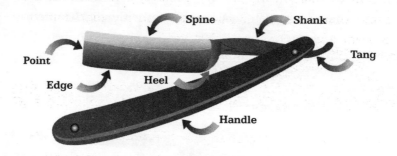

Most modern razors have a plastic handle. Some of the more expensive ones use natural buffalo horn, or exotic woods, such as desert ironwood. If it's made of wood, it's normally treated to be water-resistant. This is unnecessary because the handle of your razor should never get wet – unless, of course, you go diving at an oil-rig and find it in your back pocket. The pins that hold the razor together are not completely rust-proof, and the inside parts of the handle are difficult to dry after a shave. Therefore, the material of the handle makes no difference and comes down to pure personal choice. You can buy an antique handle on the Internet and fit it to your favourite blade. Be warned, though: this is a tricky operation.

An important thing to know about cut-throat razor blades is that most are high-carbon-content steel. For all you non-metallurgists out there, this means they're *not* stainless steel. Don't worry about this. Someone gave me a stainless-steel razor once. It's OK for what it is, but I use it now to sharpen my pencils. I simply can't achieve the same sharpness with it as I can with my high-carbon-content one, and you probably won't either.

CARING FOR YOUR CUT-THROAT RAZOR

This is crucial if you plan to use the same steel for a life-time, as I do. The best care in the world you can give your blade is to use it frequently. I've lost count of the number of razors I've seen at car-boot sales, being rained on, rust-ing. All had been sitting in a dark place, neglected, for a long time.

If you're using the blade, you'll need to dry it, strop it, and occasionally hone it, unless you're using a strop paste. Since I'm going to deal with stropping and honing in Chapter 7, I only want to mention a few essential points here. First, if you intend to leave the blade in a safe, dry place for a long time, rub it lightly with any type of machine or vegetable oil. Recently I bought razors for my two sons. I rubbed them with olive oil and put them into their boxes in a dry place. I know they'll be in perfect condition when they're needed, which will be in the distant future, since neither of my boys has started school yet. Second, when you buy a new razor, you'll notice that it's lightly covered with oil. Manufacturers know what they're doing. They know the razor may sit in a warehouse for quite a while before it's sold and used. You should therefore wash your new cut-throat razor in hot water before its first stropping: you don't want the oil to transfer itself to your strop.

The next point is of critical importance to first-time shavers. *Nearly all cut-throat razors need a light honing/ stropping before you use them.* This is regrettably true for many quality blades (but not Thiers-Issard blades). It's sad, but that's the way it is.

A brief note of caution therefore: if you're going to switch to a cut-throat razor, read Chapter 7 on honing and stropping before you proceed with your first shave. It will save you pain and heartache. Remember Toby and the grizzly bear.

That brings me to your main question: why use a cut-throat?

Most men sheer away from the very thought of a cut-throat razor. There are three main reasons they give for this:

- I don't know how to use one.
- It's dangerous: I'll cut myself badly.

- I don't have that much time to spend on shaving.

OK, let's take a closer look at these points.

I don't know how to use one.

Using a cut-throat razor is practically identical to using a safety razor. The only difference is in the grip you use. If you're using a cut-throat razor, the correct grip looks like this, with your ring finger hooked over the tang:

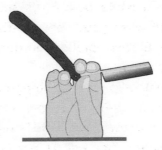

You need to remember that what you're doing is gliding a very sharp blade along your face. Well, guess what: that's exactly what you're doing when you use a safety razor.

There's also a psychological difference: when you hold a cut-throat, you are fully aware that it's a blade. A safety razor is a blade too, but it's cunningly disguised: it's encased in plastic so your instincts are fooled. My point is this: I don't want my instincts fooled. I want to know what I'm doing. I want to know I'm using a blade.

Rest assured, I've taught a couple of men how to use a cut-throat, and any man is capable of learning.

It's dangerous: I'll cut myself really badly.

You won't. You might nick yourself, but if this happens, you'll nick yourself in exactly the same way, and to the same depth, as you would with a safety razor. Remember, it's a blade, and men know how to use them. Trust me on this: you have instincts about blades, like every other man on the planet. We're not that far removed from cavemen, really.

I don't have that much time to spend on shaving.

Sadly, this is probably true. Most men don't have enough time to spend on shaving. And shaving with a cut-throat razor will take a little longer than it does with a safety. This isn't because the shave itself takes longer – in fact, a cut-throat razor is faster than a safety – but because you have to take care of the blade. It has to be honed and stropped.

But consider this: most doctors will tell you that men spend nearly every minute of their day hurtling towards a heart-attack. This is especially true of fathers and the more responsible types of middle-aged men. There's a reason we don't live into old age. Stress kills us. And I have to include myself in this group.

ENTERING THE GARDEN

Recently I went to my doctor – not for myself: two of my children needed treatment. I dressed them, gave them breakfast – none for me – fought my way through rush-hour traffic, made it into the surgery, after letting the office know I'd be late, sat, worried and comforted them in the waiting room until it was our turn. By the time we walked into the doctor's consulting room, my shirt was stuck to me with sweat and I rubbed at the stubble on my cheeks.

The doctor examined them and put my heart at ease: it was something trivial – I can't remember what. She wrote a prescription.

Then she turned to me: 'What about you?'

'Huh?'

'What about you? How are you doing?'

I had no idea how I was doing. Who cared how I was doing? Nobody ever asked me that. I was doing what I had to do, right? I was doing everything that—

'How are you doing?'

'Uuuh . . .' I stared into space, and everything went into slow-motion.

She took off her spectacles and looked at me in a kindly way. 'If you don't make time for yourself, you'll die of a heart-attack.'

I snapped out of it, of course, but later on it reminded me of something I'd read:

> Some men entering the garden begin by
> getting up at 5 a.m. and keeping an hour
> for themselves each morning before work.
> A father, in order to do that, may have to

resist his own insistence that his life belongs
to his work, his children, and his marriage.

It means that you should make time for yourself – keep it
sacred. Rushing your way through life so that you die
early isn't manly or brave. It's stupid.

Find the time to spend on your morning shave. If
you're able to arrange it so that you can shave on the
porch, or at a window overlooking your garden, so much
the better. And while you're shaving – while you're stropping and honing your blade, while you're lathering your
face – let your thoughts run in whatever direction you
like. Take the time to straighten out your head.

My final point in this chapter is concerned with something you don't need. When cut-throat razors were in
their heyday, some manufacturers came up with a great
sales pitch. They marketed the idea that you should have
a different razor for every day of the week to give the
steel time to rest between use. So, instead of selling one
blade, they could sell a set of seven. This increased sales.

It's a gimmick.

You don't need a different blade for every day of the
week, and the steel certainly doesn't need to rest. It's
probably good to have a spare, in case you damage your
blade by dropping it into the wash-basin and nicking it.
But you don't need seven. Of course, there's nothing
wrong in having seven, if you so choose. Some people

collect cut-throat razors and probably have more than a hundred. But it's not for me.

THE ONE-EYED COSSACK ✵

Quite a while ago I was in the jungle, in a bamboo hut built on stilts in northern Thailand. An open charcoal fire burned on the floor. Dawn was breaking through the trees, the sun's piercing rays hitting our faces.

There was a mixed bunch of us. I remember Nikolai, a one-eyed Cossack whose face was ravaged by loss and hardship. We'd been up all night, talking, about poetry and wars, women and God.

I saw that all the others had fallen asleep. I took out two of my last cigars (I smoke Pádrons), gave one to Nikolai and lit the second for myself. He sniffed it, rolled it between his fingers, then reached into his jacket pocket and pulled out a cut-throat razor: a Dubl Duck Wonderedge, one of the most sought-after antique blades. With it, he cut off the end of the cigar, tossed it into the fire and wiped the blade on his cuff. There was no wrapping round the razor – no case or protection.

I raised an eyebrow. 'It's a good blade.'

He nodded silently.

'You have a spare?' I asked.

I assumed, from the casual way he treated it, that he must have.

He stared into the fire, then tapped a finger against his black eye-patch. 'The man who did this to me . . .'

I waited.

He held up the razor to the light. Rays of tropical sunlight shimmered along its length. '. . . some day he will meet this razor in the dark.'

I inched away from him as he continued: 'I despise men who collect things. They're like observers in life, collecting, afraid to commit to what they have. Always looking for more.'

He pulled deep on the cigar, then hawked and spat into the fire: a sizzling sound. 'One,' he growled, 'is enough.'

Granted, this man was insane. But the fact remains that, like the one-eyed Cossack, you need only one good blade. And when you have one, you'll save a fortune in razor blades over the course of your life.

SUMMARY CHECKLIST

+ Buy a new razor.

+ Buy a Solingen or Thiers-Issard razor.

+ Wash the blade in warm water before first use.

+ Sharpen the blade before first use, unless it's a Thiers-Issard.

+ Lightly oil the blade if you're going to store it in a dry place.

+ Avoid one-eyed Cossack cigar-smokers in the jungle – they can be extremely dangerous.

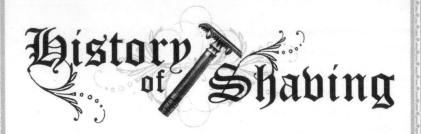 History of Shaving

THE DAWN OF MAN

It began in Africa around 100,000 BC, when cavemen started plucking out their facial hair with crude tweezers made of stone or notched seashells. At around the same time, they started painting their bodies. Until then, mankind had been quietly evolving for millions of years, and we have no idea why they suddenly started acting like this, although there have been some bizarre theories:

- That this was when we developed the tools and techniques for these activities.

- To get rid of lice and other parasites.

- To make it clear to the apes that we were different from them, and that we were in charge now.

- That we developed a higher consciousness and

invented God, which necessitated commensurate rituals.

- That planet Earth was visited by cosmonauts who were hairless and/or multicoloured and we wanted to look like them.

- That we discovered hallucinogenic plants and alcohol and lost our minds.

We do know that shaving has been connected to religious ideas since time immemorial, and still is today. Shamanism, one of the most ancient religions, regarded hair as a kind of public highway for spirits both in and out of your head. This meant that the shamanic priest doubled up as the tribal barber.

After a night of frenzied dancing, where you literally shook the bad spirits out of your free-flowing hair, the shaman would cut off your hair, so the spirits couldn't find their way back in. The shaman's hair remained long, of course, since he had lots of spirits living in there whom he needed to talk to.

Whatever the case, around 30,000 BC, men tired of plucking out their facial hairs one by one. They had invented flint blades, and could sharpen them sufficiently to shave, so that was what they started to use instead.

But flint blunts quickly. Human hair is tough. It has the same tensile strength as copper wire. Ask any barber and he'll tell you: hair wears out a lot of scissors, and plays havoc with razor blades. By the way, that's an important point to keep in mind. When you next go to shave yourself, picture your blade cutting through copper wire. Maybe then you'll be a little more thoughtful about the task you're asking your razor to perform.

But let's return to the cavemen.

Since the flint blades grew blunt so quickly, the quality of the shave was less than ideal, and they came up with the idea of dabbing on some river-mud afterwards, to ease the pain. Through trial and error, they grew to prefer those types of mud which we now know held high concentrates of vitamin A. We still use vitamin A – along with vitamin E – as a soother after shaving, and many modern aftershave balms rely on it.

But the mud introduced a new dimension. A few hours later when it was washed off, dark lines sometimes appeared where the user had cut himself, since many types of mud contain powerful natural dyes. So, along with shaving, cavemen had invented the art of facial tattooing – two traditions that would, somewhat bizarrely, continue side by side for a few thousand years. Wavy lines and spirals were quite a common sight on the faces of our cave-dwelling ancestors, as they are with the Maori to this day.

Soon after the introduction of flint, some started using sharpened seashells as blades, but the idea never caught on, and it was only in 3000 BC, when mankind invented metalworking, that flint had a serious rival.

At around this time, we find copper-alloy razors being used in ancient India and Egypt. And it was in Egypt, as we will see later, that things started to become interesting on the shaving front.

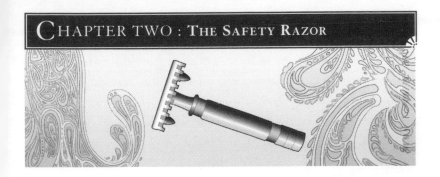

CHAPTER TWO : THE SAFETY RAZOR

I t was a winter's morning of my childhood. The hoar-frost lay thick on the grass, and my breath formed puffs of cloud. I was running down to Great-uncle Hector's house to borrow a bag of sugar for my mum. There were no twenty-four-hour, seven-days-a-week convenience shops then. It was a Sunday, and if you hadn't bought it during the week, you waited until Monday.

I tore up the gravelled driveway, rang the bell, and heard Great-aunt Genevieve shuffling down the hall, opening the heavy door, with the stained glass. She was all slippers and warm smiles. 'He's just starting, lad.'

I raced up the stairs, turning to shout back at her from the landing: 'Mum needs to borrow some sugar.'

I hurtled down the hall in a few steps, and then I was in the washroom, and there was Great-uncle Hector, gazing out of the window with a mournful eye.

Looking back, I didn't know much about Great-uncle Hector, but what I did know fixed him firmly in my head as the kind of man I wanted to be. I knew he'd been shot in the stomach in Spain, fighting against Franco, and that he'd also been shot in the arse by a jealous husband. He'd travelled by steamer to Brazil, and had lived in the jungle there with real Indians. He had a pair of cavalry sabres hanging on his study wall, and a brace of antique pistols. It was darkly rumoured that he had a loaded revolver stashed somewhere in the house, and that Great-aunt Genevieve was constantly on the lookout for it, to hand it in to the police.

One of the things I remember most clearly is his shaving room – the washroom: high-ceilinged, with a red-and-black-tiled floor, oak-panelled walls, musty old coats and paintings leaning here and there, and a stag's head mounted high, staring with vacant eyes. Great-uncle Hector's three separate strops hung from the various points of its antlers. He had an old Belfast sink under the window, and a whistling kettle on a gas-burner beside it, so that when he shaved, he looked out of the window on to his garden: at the cherry and apple trees he had planted, and his vegetable plot, where carrots and lettuces grew, rhododendrons and irises, and a lawn that stretched for ever. Here, he watched the seasons turn, and let his thoughts wander through the corridors of his memory.

On days when there was no school, I was allowed to sit there, on the windowsill, as he stropped and shaved and told me about the Indians and his vegetables and the time he was shot by the Fascists. He always refused to discuss the jealous husband.

I'd rarely seen Great-uncle Hector look mournful, so I knew something was up.

'Hello, lad.'

I stared at him or, more specifically, at what he had in his hand. The cut-throat that I knew so well was gone. In its place was an unlooked-for piece of steel, shaped like a small hoe.

'It's a safety razor, lad. Doctor's orders, I'm afraid.'

He raised his hand to hold it level with his eyes, and as he held it there, I noticed for the first time how old he was. His hand shook like a leaf.

'You know, lad, if I'd had hands like this back then, I never would've been able to hold my gun against the Fascists.' He smiled at my consternation. 'But progress is a great thing. Look, I'll be able to shave myself like a gentleman for another good few years.'

And he did. To his dying day, I never saw Great-uncle Hector with stubble on his cheeks.

So, no, I'm not one of those zealots who believe that anyone who doesn't use a cut-throat razor is damned for all eternity. Each to his own, I say, and I acknowledge that the majority of people who shave nowadays, in the West, use a safety razor.

Even back then Great-uncle Hector was something of an anachronism as regards his choice of shaving technology. The hoe-type razor was invented in 1847 by an Englishman called William Henson. The British army – in contrast to the American – continued to use the cut-throat razor during the First World War. But by 1920 even they had converted to the safety razor.

I myself used a safety for years before switching to a cut-throat, and recently – by way of research for this book – I've been using a safety now and then, taking notes on its performance for your exclusive benefit.

So here you go.

DISPOSABLE-BLADE RAZORS

The original safety razor – the one that displaced the cut-throat – was still an all-metal tool. You had a holder, which could be in itself a work of art. Some were gold-plated, with beautiful designs etched in. And you fixed the disposable blade into it. The blade was two-sided, which was handy, and you had a wide choice of brands to choose from.

The original big seller was, of course, Gillette. These blades were easily recognizable by virtue of the fact that their packaging all carried Mr Gillette's picture. Even in the remotest jungle outpost, tribesmen would barter for razor blades 'with the picture of the white man'.

But everyone had his favourite blade, and you were spoiled for choice. The real determining factor was how long your blade lasted before you had to swap it for a new one.

That was where Wilkinson Sword came in. In the

1960s, they started making their disposable blade with stainless steel and launched their marketing campaign: they claimed it lasted five times longer than other blades. Soon they were one of the world leaders and, of course, the other companies started using stainless steel too.

Incidentally, the Wilkinson Sword company also launched the marketing campaign that told American women to shave their armpits: underarm hair was unfeminine and unhygienic.

As for the performance of disposable blades, I have to say this: the old-fashioned, insert-a-blade safety razor works fine. Great-uncle Hector grew quite fond of his, although he gazed longingly at his strops every now and then. I've tested a few in my day, and I've no complaints as regards closeness of shave, as long as you have a modicum of technique to go with it. Also, these razors can make shaving a more personal activity than the current disposable cartridge razors. If you're one of those men who prefer old to new and craftsmanship to technology, you should test-drive one.

The principal advantage of the old-fashioned disposable-blade safety razors is that they're cheap. In their heyday, everyone used one. Now, no one does. You can find them floating around flea-markets, car-boot sales, or on the Internet for next to nothing. Even better: buy one in an exotic location and let it remind you of it every time you shave. They can be a lot of fun.

As for the blades: they won't set you back much. In

the long run, your wallet will definitely thank you for switching from a disposable cartridge razor to this type.

There is one final point I'd like to mention in connection with the disposable-blade safety razor: it's worthwhile finding yourself a container for the used blades instead of discarding them one by one. (Great-uncle Hector used an old jam-jar.) The discarded blades used to cause quite a few accidents involving binmen's hands in their day, and they're still a serious hazard if not kept safe. When they go into the bin, they should be safely housed in a non-pierceable container such as stiff cardboard or plastic.

CARTRIDGE RAZORS

Lots of older men still use the original safety razors, but you only have to visit your local supermarket – the men's shaving section – to realize that this way of shaving is on the way out. You'll see that one or two inches of the display are devoted to these blades, and the rest of the shelf is taken up with strange plastic contraptions. The disposable cartridge razor, of which the Gillette Mach 3 is the dominant brand, has taken the bulk of the market.

The cartridge razor emerged in the late 1960s. It's basically a plastic cartridge, containing one, two or three blades that you insert into a handle, which can be steel, plastic or even solid gold. It has many variations, swivel-head, lubri-strip and injectors being the most common.

Swivel-heads were clever. Your guiding hand didn't need to be in tune with every bump and curve on your face: the cartridge swivelled round them, keeping the blade close to your skin, which equated with a closer shave and fewer cuts. In theory, it eliminates amateurs digging away at those tough-to-reach areas and giving themselves razor-burn.

On the other hand, I always found the lubri-strip dubious. It presupposed that your lather was in some way deficient, or that you hadn't applied it correctly (actually, those are two accurate presuppositions with most men), so took care of it for you by lubricating the area immediately in front of the blade. I suppose it's a nice theory, but I always found it annoying. Then again, I trust my shaving soap and lathering technique.

PLASTIC THROWAWAYS

The simplest safety razor – and the one I started with before that disastrous school disco – was a plastic throwaway. One blade, no cartridge, no lubri-strip, no swivel-head, no fancy gadgets. They are still available, and in the interests of a trip down Memory Lane, I bought one recently and used it.

It works fine, albeit I found myself making shorter, choppier strokes with it than I would with my cut-throat. But there was no razor-burn or nick. I used it four times in four days, and it still held true. I remember in my younger years I used them for far longer than that. There were times when I had a blade on the go for months, but this isn't something I'd recommend.

THE TWIN BLADE

The single blade was a functional piece of technology if ever there was one. But then they went and invented the twin-blade. 'Big deal,' you say. 'Why don't you simply go over it twice with the single blade?' The answer is, no, it's not the same. Here's the theory.

The first blade, as it cuts, also pulls the hair slightly out of its follicle. Before that hair can retract back into the follicle, the second blade comes along and, *whack!*, slices another bit off, so that when the hair does retract into the follicle, it will be beneath the surface of the skin. This should give you a face as smooth as a baby's bottom. This theory is called 'hysteresis'.

Does it work?

I'll have to borrow Carl R. Rogers's answer to that:

> Neither the Bible nor the prophets –
> neither Freud nor research – neither the
> revelations of God nor man – can take
> precedence over my own direct
> experience.

Who am I to tell you to use one blade, two or three? My overriding central philosophy, as regards shaving at any rate, is to try it and see if it works for you. If you've been using a single-blade razor, why not try a twin-blade? I find a twin-blade gives me a similar shave to a single-blade, although certainly not as smooth a shave as a cut-throat. If you like the twin-blade, you can stick with it. If not, you haven't lost much, have you?

So now you're wondering: hey, if that theory works for two blades, then maybe . . .

THE MACH 3

I remember when the Mach 3 was launched. I was sitting in front of the TV. I can't remember what I was watching, but let's pretend it was *The Godfather* (because I like it). I picked up a book during the ads. But I was interrupted by the roar of a jet. It was a powerful, sexy-sounding jet, of the kind featured in *Top Gun*, and I dropped my book to see what on earth they were trying to sell me.

A razor?

But not just any razor: it was the birth of Mach 3. They had a man on there who looked rugged and handsome, and that blade – or, rather, those three blades – were gliding across his face in the same way that the jet was gliding across the skies. If I recall correctly, the ad featured a woman's hands gliding across his face too.

It was powerful stuff, especially if you were a teenager hankering after those hands – which, let's face it, we all were.

The time was ripe for it. The great lumbering mass of Western manhood migrated to the Mach 3, and Gillette made a fortune.

Not out of me, though. I stuck with my plastic single-blade disposables, which I continued to use for months on end before replacing them. I was a stubborn, ignorant individual even then.

But I bought a Mach 3 recently, test-drove it several times, and here's the verdict.

It's a cartridge razor, with a swivel-head and three blades so, in theory, the hysteresis effect should work twice, and your face should be very smooth indeed. I should note also that the one I bought had a variation of the lubri-strip in reverse: more a kind of soothing strip. It's a green strip containing aloe vera and vitamin E that glides over your face after the blades. Aloe vera is a great soother, as anyone who's experienced sunburn will know. And vitamin E has all kinds of regenerative properties that work well on freshly shaven skin. The green strip turns white when it's time for you to change the blade – a handy little indicator.

Again, you ask, does it work? Is it worth the money? Well, it worked fine for me. There were no ill-effects, no razor-burn or blood. The shave was smooth, but no smoother than that of the cheap plastic disposable – at least, not that my fingers could detect.

Which brings me to the question of skill and the acceptance of new technology. And we're going to have to revisit Great-uncle Hector for this one since he had the age and experience to be able to answer such a thorny question.

LUDDITES

Winter had passed, and the cherry blossom was out. The smell of mown grass hung in the air, and filled the wash-room. I was watching Great-uncle Hector go through his morning ritual. He was quite proficient with the safety razor by then and there were quite a few used blades in his jam-jar.

He paused in the middle of a stroke and lifted the razor to the light, squinting at it. 'You know they're using electric shavers now, lad.'

I nodded. I had heard of them. In fact, my cousin used one.

He rinsed the blade in the basin. 'There's nothing wrong with this razor. I've grown to quite like the little gadget. And, I confess, I hated it at first. But it's not doing anyone any harm, now, is it?'

'Course not, Uncle Hector.'

'Exactly, lad. Exactly.'

I scratched my head.

He sighed and stared out at the cherry blossom. 'Your great-aunt Genevieve wants me to switch to an electric, lad.'

I waited.

'I can't do it, lad – just can't do it. I've too much of the Luddite in me. I'm too bloody old to have an electric engine crawling all over my face. Next thing you know, the scientists will have us shooting our beards off with bloody laser beams.'

Great-uncle Hector never did go electric, despite Great-aunt Genevieve's best efforts. He came to know his safety razor well and was thankful for it, but enough was enough.

There's probably a good deal of the Luddite in me too. I can see the point in having a safety razor, and I can see the point in the twin-blade, since hysteresis seems like a solid theory. But I'm not sure I need three or four blades 'crawling over my face', doing the job that one blade can do equally well.

SHAVING IN THE SHOWER

Some men really like shaving in the shower. If this is for you, then the safety razor is the one to go with. You should never, ever, use a cut-throat in the shower. First, it will be ruined in quite a short time. But also, if you drop it, you could ruin a damn sight more than the razor.

If you're shaving in the shower, it's probably worthwhile investing in a non-fogging mirror to do away with all that tedious wiping. They are normally made of acrylics. In some, the hot water is pumped through the back of the mirror; others have a heating pad. (Condensation forms when there's a variation in temperature on two sides of the glass.)

There's a lot to be said for shaving in the shower. It makes rinsing easier. The steam is good for softening those bristles and, importantly, you're generally undisturbed in there. The only piece of advice I'll give is this: don't get carried away.

LIAM'S WILD SIDE

A friend of mine, Liam, used to shave in the shower. He was a tough guy. He didn't have to pretend like the rest of us. He was a hard-core rugby player, and he really enjoyed it. Crashing into people at full speed and trampling them into the mud was his idea of wholesome fun.

One day, as we were changing to troop out for a game, I noticed something odd about him.

'Wha' . . . ?'

He dropped his head and pulled on his shirt fast. 'I shaved.'

'Your chest?'

'Yeah. I didn't really mean to. I got carried away. I was in the shower, and I just kind of . . . I think I would have shaved my legs if I hadn't run out of hot water. I don't know what came over me.'

Now, if a morally upstanding rugby player like Liam, who later became a bank manager, can do that kind of thing, what hope is there for the rest of us?

Men do strange things in the shower, given the opportunity.

THE SHAPE OF THINGS TO COME

There's only one thing left to discuss as regards the safety razor, and that's the future.

At the moment, the great mass of Western manhood is using the Mach 3 or similar. That represents a lot of money for the shaving companies, especially the large ones.

I've been employed by some major multinationals in my time, and as a result, I understand a bit about the way they operate. One thing they need to do is to keep improving, because if they don't, other companies will swallow them. You could compare it to a fish-tank, with the meaner fish eating the lazier ones. To stay ahead of the pack, you keep bringing out new products, even if the old ones are good enough.

So, even though people seemed happy with one blade, the shaving companies brought out the twin-blade, then the Mach 3, and you can buy razors now with four blades

– the Quattro – and guess what: I've seen the future, and it's five blades.

My God! Five?

Five, with the blades spaced far closer together than they are currently. This will form a kind of shaving surface instead of a strip, which will probably be good for shaving large flat areas, like your cheeks. But it's going to be hell shaving in the confined space under your nose. In fact, that's one of the biggest complaints about the Mach 3: you can't travel close enough to your nose when shaving the upper lip. So, on the next generation, they have a single blade on the reverse side of the head to allow you to get closer to your nose, and to enable you to give yourself an accurate trim on your sideburns. That's a good idea.

Those razors also contain a microchip, and a battery. Here's how they work. When you start your shave, you switch the razor on, and the microchip sends – or, rather, regulates – a series of micro-pulses down to the blades. As a micro-pulse is a tiny vibration, you now have a vibrating blade.

Wow! Will it work?

When it comes out, why don't you try it and see?

As for me, it's a little too close to shooting my beard off with bloody laser beams. I take my hat off to Great-uncle Hector.

SUMMARY CHECKLIST

✦ Experiment. Try them all and settle for the one that suits you.

✦ Disposable blades are cheaper in the long run. The razor can also become a personal belonging.

✦ Multiple-blade safety razors are good on flat surfaces, like your cheeks, but can be awkward in other areas, like the upper lip.

✦ Shaving in the shower is fun. Try it and see if it works for you.

✦ Take comfort from the fact that even the most upstanding citizen you know has probably, at some point in his life, taken a walk on the wild side.

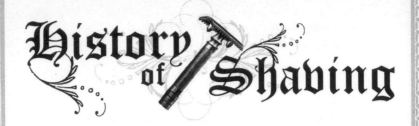

History of Shaving

ANCIENT EGYPT

The ancient Egyptians took shaving to a new level. It wasn't only about facial hair any more: head, face, eyebrows, legs, chest and unmentionable parts all went under the razor, for men, women and children.

In the early days of the Old Kingdom, they used copper blades. Then, between 1567 and 1320 BC, they switched to bronze – a big step forward in metallurgy. Egyptian razors were hatchet-shaped affairs, with curved handles. They also used pumice stones, tweezers and depilatory creams made of arsenic, quicklime and starch to eliminate body hair.

Not all of Egyptian society shaved, of course. Peasants, mercenaries, criminals, barbarians (i.e. foreigners) and plunderers wore beards. Facial hair was an instant indicator of class.

In the interest of dignity, sometimes nobles and priests felt the need of a beard. At those times, they strapped on an artificial, metal one. But, as a general rule, the higher you ascended on the social ladder, the more diligent you were about washing and shaving. The Egyptian nobility bathed themselves upwards of three times daily, and their priests were required to shave themselves all over at least every third day.

There were, of course, practical reasons for this. Egypt was, and remains, a swelteringly hot country, and shampoo was unknown. Long, dirty hair in a hot climate makes for lice, which were practically impossible to avoid – hence the all-over shaving routine. But since a bald head in a sweltering hot country also equates to sunstroke, they made wigs for themselves. And the wigs they designed were advanced solar-protection units. They protruded out to provide cover to the neck and face in ways that natural hair could never do. Shaving (and the accompanying wigs) was a clever adaptation to the climate.

So in many ways shaving was the defining Egyptian trait, and this could generate conflict when challenged, most famously by the Israelites and their leader.

MOSES

Most people have Moses fixed in their mind as a bearded patriarch, which was what he became in later years. But you must remember that he had been raised in the royal palace alongside Pharaoh, and in his youth he would have been as clean-shaven as the rest of the nobility.

But when Moses appeared before the pharaoh of his day (possibly, but not certainly, Ramses II), telling him to let his people go, he did so wearing long hair and a full beard. This was asking for trouble. Everyone shaved before they appeared before Pharaoh. Even the Israelite Joseph, of amazing technicolour dreamcoat fame, had been shaved before he went to see him. Moses demanding the emancipation of his nation was one thing, but the beard was the final straw. Predictably, things took a bad turn, what with the plagues, and armies of chariots being smashed to the bottom of the Red Sea. But Moses came through it all with his beard intact.

After Moses, the bearded patriarch became the vogue. People started to attach undue importance to facial hair. A whole new dimension was introduced into shaving. It wasn't about personal preference any more, or even about hygiene. Religion took over, with instructions such as those below:

- *Islam*. 'Trim closely the moustache, and grow the beard, and thus act against the fire-worshippers.'

- *Buddhism*. 'The shaving of the hair symbolizes renunciation and marks one's departure from the worldly life. Thus monks are advised to shave and keep the hair short.'

- *Judaism*. 'Do not cut the hair at the sides of your head or clip off the edges of your beard.'

- *Christianity*. 'For God wished women to be smooth and to rejoice in their locks alone growing spontaneously, as a horse in his mane. But he adorned man like the lions, with a beard, and endowed him, as an attribute of manhood, with a hairy chest – a sign of strength and rule.'

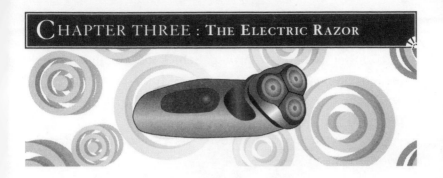

In the year 1910, in Alaska, a Mr Jacob Schick sat in a tent in the middle of nowhere. He was one of those men in history who like doing things their own way.

When he was a young man, Schick joined the army. After contracting dysentery in the Philippines, a some-what deranged army doctor suggested his health would improve if he transferred to Alaska. After a few years there, Schick decided to retire from military service and do some prospecting for gold in the wilderness. And that was how he came to be sitting in that tent in the middle of nowhere.

The temperature was somewhere around minus 40 degrees Fahrenheit. And Schick was confined to camp because he had sprained his ankle.

Apart from the cold, his biggest problem was his diet. He had shot a moose a few days previously, and it was moose for breakfast, lunch and dinner. The moose carcass was frozen solid. Whenever he felt hungry, he'd hack a piece off with a hatchet and cook it over the campfire. He had tried it boiled, fried and roasted, but there was no disguising the essential taste of moose.

On that particular morning, Schick looked out over the leaden sky, trying to make out the horizon, but after a while he gave up. Everything seemed grey, even the heavy flakes that drifted down around him.

He rubbed his fingers over his cheeks, and decided two things:

- He was going to skip the moose breakfast.
- He was going to shave.

He hobbled over to a rain barrel and, with an ice-pick, jabbed at it until he had a couple of ice-chunks as big as his fist. He dropped them into a pan, then balanced it on the campfire.

The campfire wasn't warm enough to melt the ice, so he had to collect some more branches and twigs to build it up. But before he put the branches on to the fire, he had to brush the snow off them, and knock some ice off too, since it would have put out the fire as it melted. After a few minutes of this his fingers went numb.

Finally, he carried a pot of tepid water back to the tent, slopping some on his shoes. His sprained ankle meant he had to hobble, and every step sent waves of pain into his head.

At the entrance, he paused at the half-eaten moose. It looked like something from the Apocalypse. He cursed silently and squeezed past it into the tent. He unpacked his shaving gear, inserted a fresh blade into his safety razor, and started to lather up with the melted water.

He managed that all right, but when it came to the shave, his fingers let him down. They were frozen. He tried everything to breathe life back into them, but in the end he had to start the shave fast, before the water froze too.

It was a lousy shave – maybe his worst ever. He cut himself, and there were uneven, stubbly patches, and areas where he was rubbed raw.

'Dammit all to hell!'

He threw the razor in the general direction of the water, which was a big mistake. It hit the pot and knocked it over. Even as he watched in horror, the steam from the warm water disappeared as it froze in a layer over his blankets and clothes.

He rubbed his eyes in a defeated way. The whole process was wrong. It was unbelievable that men in this enlightened age were still using primitive blades to remove their facial hair. It was unbelievable how cold Alaska was. Most of all, it was unbelievable that he had eaten nothing but moose for an entire week.

'There must be a better way.'

He thought about this a little. Then he squared his shoulders. Not for nothing had he been a first lieutenant of the Alaskan 22nd Infantry Regiment.

'If there isn't a better way, I'm going to invent one. There should be a machine.' He picked up the razor and glowered at it. 'I'm going to invent a machine. A shaving machine. There'll be an engine and everything. Electricity. That's what I'll use.'

He glared at his shaving brush, and then at the water, now ice, splashed around the tent.

'And, what's more, there'll be no more need for water, or brushes, or lather, or soap, or blades, or anything like that. It's going to be an electric shaver that you can use without anything else. It'll be convenient and clean and not messy. That's right – and I'll call it the electric razor, because that's what it's going to be.'

So First Lieutenant Jacob Schick, in the Alaskan wilderness, took out a pen and paper and invented the electric razor.

It wasn't all plain sailing, of course. There were interruptions. The First World War took up a lot of his time: he re-enlisted and went to England, where he was put in charge of troop movement. He was also promoted to lieutenant colonel.

But he couldn't put the electric shaver out of his mind, and when he finally left the army, he followed through on his idea, making prototypes, starting a company and building up finance. Finally, he introduced the first usable electric razors to the market. People liked the idea and bought them. The electric razor was here to stay.

Today 30 per cent of all the men who shave in the UK use an electric razor. Its advantages are obvious:

- It's fast.
- It's simple: a child, or a teenager, can use one.
- You can do it in the car while you're stuck in traffic on the way to work.
- You probably won't damage yourself.
- You'll save money in the long run, assuming that you use your electric razor for any length of time.

So why only 30 per cent? Why not everyone?
Because there are disadvantages too:

- There's an initial capital investment that's beyond the reach of quite a few teenagers.
- Some people maintain that it doesn't give you as smooth a shave as a blade – in fact, there's considerable debate about this.
- The first time round, it's not as exciting as using a real blade on your face.
- It may irritate, or inflame, your skin more than a wet shave.
- Initially, there may be some discomfort when you're using it.

The Adjustment Period

That last point about discomfort: I can state, from first-hand experience, that it's true. I started shaving with a disposable, which I've talked about already, and then I moved on to a cut-throat. But a few years ago, I decided to buy an electric razor so that in an emergency (my life is full of emergencies) I could shave fast before I had to be somewhere important. I thought that an electric might be handy and, because I believe in quality, I bought an expensive one.

I used it twice, then threw it into the bin. I couldn't take the pain. I swear it felt as if my bristles were being yanked out one by one. The manufacturers admit this: they state openly that an 'adjustment period', or 'adequate trial period', is required. It normally lasts about thirty days.

So that's something to bear in mind if you're thinking about an electric razor. If switching is important to you – as it obviously wasn't to me – go through with the trial period and make your judgement then. And during this trial period, don't jump back and forth between a wet shave and an electric one, or you'll never get used to it.

OSCILLATING AND ROTARY RAZORS

There are fundamentally two types of electric razor: the rotary action, and the oscillating/vibrating action.

Rotary-action shavers are easy to recognize: they have little roundy bits on the head, which do the shaving. There are normally three roundy bits, although you can buy razors with two.

Inside those roundy bits is a bushel of tiny blades that rotate at high speed. There's a protective foil above the blades – otherwise they would dig into your skin, causing massive blood-loss and extreme pain. Your stubble pokes through the openings in the protective barrier and is lopped off by the rotating blades.

Oscillating shavers have a curved head with a protective foil covering. Inside the foil are lots of blades that move from side to side (oscillating means 'going back and forth'). Again, your stubble pokes through the tiny openings in the protective foil and the blades go to work on it. There are oscillating razors with only one row of blades under a foil. Then there are razors with two or three foils and the equivalent rows of blades. Hence we talk about single foil, double foil, triple foil, etc.

The traditional theory on electric razors is this: when you're using an electric shaver, your stubble should stand straight and firm. That will make it easier for it to poke through the protective foil, and thus easier for those tiny, extremely fast blades to cut them off.

You can compare an electric razor to a lawnmower. Anyone who's ever mown a lawn knows that you do it when the grass is dry, and therefore standing upright, and it's the same with electric razors.

So it's the opposite to wet-shaving, when your stubble should be as soft and pliable as possible. That's why, if you use an electric razor, you should shave before you have a shower. You can purchase pre-shave lotions designed to dry the oils and moisture on your stubble, to make it stand upright. Many are alcohol-based, since alcohol is great for clearing oil. The problem, of course, is that alcohol can irritate your skin, so it may be worth trying one that's alcohol-free.

But just when everything seemed so straightforward, they changed the game. There are models on sale now that contain an integrated capsule or sachet that dispenses lotion or gel on to your skin. And they score quite well in independent evaluations – men like them.

If you decide to go for one of these models, you should try both the lotion and gel options and see which works best for you. Key words to look out for are 'vitamin-enriched', and 'alcohol-free'. Incidentally, the sachets they sell with the razor can easily be filled with your favourite brand of lotion or gel, which may work out cheaper. Given that the gel will have practically zero time to soften the stubble, the main benefit you're left with is lubrication.

I confess that I've never used one. My only experience with an electric razor was enough to last me a lifetime. The theory isn't that difficult, though: you press a little button and a small quantity of gel squeezes out. Then you use the razor head to rub it in as the blades cut through the stubble.

They've started putting a range of additional features on electric shavers now that can be bewildering for the beginner.

You can buy models with 'gears' so you can increase the RPMs (rotations per minute) at which your blades whirl round. If you're one of those men who always wanted that stick-shift convertible, but never managed it, then this feature is for you. As you move up a gear to take out the really tough stubble on your chin, close your eyes and picture yourself as James Bond outmanoeuvring the villains in his customized Aston Martin.

However, if you're the type who gets excited about the latest technologies, you should invest in a model with an LCD screen. LCD stands for 'liquid crystal display', which in itself is a nice piece of technology – although, to be honest, it's old hat at this stage of the game.

LCDs are basically a thin film of twisted crystals with polarizing filters on either side. Some of the crystals are hit with an electric charge, which 'untwists' them and stops the light passing through. The ones that aren't electrically charged remain twisted and continue to allow the light to pass through. The darker numbers on your LCD are therefore electrically charged crystals.

So now you know.

LCDs are in widespread use everywhere. Electric razors include them mostly to tell you how much time is left in your battery. That can be useful, I suppose. Other models simply incorporate a red light that flashes on when it's time to recharge and does the job just as well. The term 'over-engineering' might be relevant here – it's one of my favourites.

While I'm on the subject of batteries, here's some interesting back-pocket information. Again, like LCDs, this information is relevant to more than electric razors:

- *NiCd (nickel cadmium)* batteries contain cadmium, which is harmful to the environment, so you should dispose of them carefully. These are the original, reliable, rechargeable batteries.
- *NiMH (nickel-metal hydride)* batteries are a more recent arrival. They're generally more powerful than NiCd batteries and less harmful to the environment.
- *LiIon (lithium-ion)* batteries are the latest thing. They have higher capacity, and they're much faster to recharge. They're expensive, though.

So, instead of asking the shop assistant for a new battery for your digital watch, you can ask him for a lithium-ion battery. You'll probably find he won't know what you're talking about. Three-quarters of technical knowledge is being familiar with the vocabulary.

One practical thing you should take into consideration when buying an electric shaver is whether it has a built-in voltage converter. If you're a frequent traveller to a country that uses a different voltage from your own, it's worth spending the money. True, you can buy external converters, but they tend to be bulky.

Another gadget that's probably worth having on your electric razor is a beard-trimmer. This looks and works like a miniature hair-clipper. It's handy for edging that straight line on your sideburns, or if you intend to do any fancy work, as in zigzag lines.

It can also be useful – although it's not strictly intended for this – for cutting down long stubble if you haven't shaved for a while.

If you can compare the electric razor to a lawnmower, then the beard-trimmer is a scythe, for that very long grass.

THE HAIR-CLIPPER

The barber's essential tool for the crew-cut look. A lot of men have one at home now. I have a hair-clipper: every so often I take my hair down to about half an inch. If your stubble has gone completely out of control, a disposable razor, like a Mach 3, will get lost in it, and an electric shaver will become clogged. You'll either have to take scissors to it or use a hair-clipper, and a hair-clipper is a lot faster and more convenient.

My first experience with a hair-clipper was in Abu

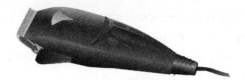

Dhabi. I arrived with very long hair, but soon discovered the heat. I'm not talking about the everyday heat we experience in the temperate climate of Europe or North America. This heat was like a living thing. After the ten-minute walk to my school (I was teaching) my hair was dripping. I grew tired of it very quickly.

My flatmate was a Scot, with very short hair indeed, and he had a hair-clipper that he let me borrow. After using it a few times, I decided to buy my own and found one in the local *souk* – the market.

It was incredibly cheap, but what surprised me most was the strength of the engine. It must have had two or three times the power of my Scottish flatmate's. Soon he was using mine too, and we developed a routine of clipping each other's hair every couple of weeks.

When I left Abu Dhabi, I knew I was going to grow my hair again, and I didn't want the clipper, so I gave it to my flatmate. As I was looking it over one last time, I noticed some fine print near the power flex.

'For livestock only. Unsuitable for human use.'

We'd been using sheep shears on our heads all year.

Let's return to electric razors.

Some electric razors can be used in the shower, or the

bath, if that's what you want. Some have an anti-slip grip. There are razors with pivot heads, fixed heads and individually floating heads. These features all serve to keep the shave close, but not too close.

There are razors with lift-and-cut technology, and something called 'smart foil', which means that the foil has different-sized and -shaped holes, scientifically designed to catch even the most stubborn facial hair.

There are razors with a hair-collection chamber, which sounds useful, and there are razors with a jet-clean system, and about every other kind of self-cleaning system you can think of. Some come with dinky little brushes for cleaning out the hair. Others have shaving heads that are designed to be held under the tap and rinsed, which might be worth paying extra for.

While I'm on the subject of cleaning, most manufacturers are very clear that you shouldn't knock the electric razor against the side of the wash-basin to clean out the hair. Notwithstanding this, that's exactly what a lot of men do. Those who don't normally blow into it. I confess, when I'm cleaning my electric clipper, I'm tempted to do both, but I stop myself.

Knocking a machine with moving parts against a solid object is – from a mechanical point of view – galactically stupid. Blowing into a finely tuned piece of machinery is also wrong: no matter how hard you try not to, you will spit into it. Even if your breath feels perfectly dry, there are little bits of spit in there. It's not a good idea. Use the little brush they sold you with the shaver, and while you're at it, read the manual.

COST

The determining factor with the electric razor is its price. With a disposable safety razor, you can try out many models and settle on the one you like best. Disposable razors are cheap.

With an electric razor, you're stuck with the one you buy, or the one your parents bought you when you were a teenager. Most men won't buy another electric razor if they have a functioning one at home.

Therefore, when you buy one, take your time. Go to a shop with a wide selection where the assistants have been trained in the technology. The last thing you want to hear when you ask about a built-in voltage converter is 'Huh?'

Go with the best model you can afford. You'll be using that razor for a long time to come.

So, now you're holding your electric razor: how do you use it?

I have exactly two tips about the actual process of shaving with an electric razor.

First, don't press the head hard into your skin. You can give yourself razor-burn with an electric razor, exactly as you can with a blade. It should rest lightly on the surface.

Second, you might want to consider shaving the sensitive areas first, before the razor head has time to heat up and cause irritation.

Here's your technique: you run it over your face, again and again, until it feels smooth enough to stop. It's not hard. In fact, it's exactly what Mr Jacob Schick had in mind in that tent in Alaska.

SUMMARY CHECKLIST

✢ If you're going to use an electric razor, it's worthwhile going upmarket, since you're probably not going to upgrade any time soon.

✢ Unless your electric razor has a gel-dispensing function built into it, shave before you have a shower.

✢ If you're determined to switch from a wet shave to an electric razor, give yourself about a month to acclimatize.

✢ If your doctor tells you to move to Alaska for health reasons, find yourself a new doctor.

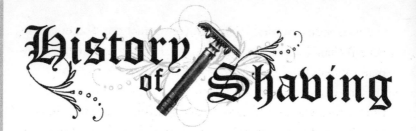

History of Shaving

THE GREEKS

The ancient Greeks wore spectacular beards and spent a lot of time having them oiled and curled by their local barber. The quality of a man's beard was important. When Socrates was brought to trial on a charge of corrupting Athenian youth, one of his accusers, Meletus, was described as having a beak, long straight hair and an ill-grown beard. After Socrates committed suicide, Meletus was himself accused and executed. The ill-grown beard probably didn't help.

All of this changed with Alexander the Great. He was one of the most handsome men of the age, and possibly for this reason he held with the clean-shaven look. He was very particular about it, absolutely refusing to go into battle with five o'clock shadow. Some people say it was because he was homosexual, but really that's neither here nor there.

The thing was, he expected his army to follow suit. In the middle of his massive war against the Persians (also bearded), one of his officers came to him and told him that everything was prepared for the upcoming battle, and did he require anything further?

Alexander replied: 'Nothing, but that the Macedonians cut off their beards, for there is not a better handle to take a man by than the beard.'

But Alexander was up against centuries of male tradition. There was an old Greek saying: 'There are two kinds of people in this world who go around beardless, boys and women, and I am neither one.'

So the men were reluctant and, accordingly, they went into battle wearing their beards.

As it happened, that battle turned into a horrific mess, and in the middle of it, quite close to Alexander, a Greek officer named Philip was grabbed by the beard. As he winced and struggled, the Persian warrior drew an enormous sword and whacked his head clean off. Not content with that, the Persian then hurled the severed head straight at Alexander, narrowly missing him.

Alexander was incandescent with rage. The next day, he had his men lined up in the midday sun, and when he had their attention, he produced Philip's head from a bag and held it high so they could all take a good look.

'You all remember Philip, I presume?'

The men muttered and shuffled.

'Take a closer look, then.' Alexander whirled the head round in an arc and fired it into the ranks. It ricocheted off someone's helmet with a clang, then rolled to a stop in the dust. The Macedonians were outraged, and some wondered if their general wasn't losing his marbles.

'Philip would be alive today if he had shaved, as I clearly

ordered. We nearly lost that battle, and next time round, the first man I see wearing a beard will be stationed a hundred paces to the front of the phalanx.'

There was grumbling, of course, and some of the more traditional men still refused, but the bulk of the army shaved: anyone standing that far ahead of the phalanx was a goner for sure. And, clean-shaven, they went on to conquer the Persian Empire as far as India.

When he returned from India, Alexander became a little unstable and drank himself to death. But his legacy lived on: his victorious army kept up the shaving, and it was only a matter of time before the civilian population followed suit – since time immemorial, the military has set the fashion in matters of facial hair. Shaving spread rapidly throughout Macedonia and Greece and, importantly, to the Greek colonies in southern Italy.

The Greek women were surprised by this turn of events, but not altogether displeased. To repay the favour to their men, they took to singeing the hair off their legs with oil lamps.

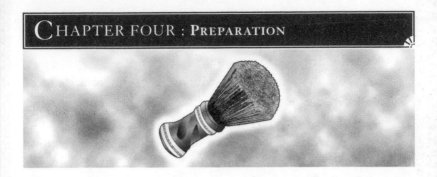

Prince Otto Eduard Leopold von Bismarck – the Iron Chancellor of Prussia – stood in front of an enormous wall-map of France. He whacked it angrily with a stick, leaving a dent over Paris. 'France.'

The other man in the room, Helmuth Karl Bernhard, Graf von Moltke, nodded. 'Yes, Chancellor.'

Bismarck whacked the map again. 'The question is, do you have a battle-plan that will defeat the French?'

Moltke shrugged. 'No battle-plan survives contact with the enemy. It's the central point of my entire philosophy.'

Bismarck scowled. He wondered sometimes if Moltke wasn't a little too clever for his boots. 'Are we prepared for war, Moltke? Is the Prussian army prepared? Are you yourself prepared?'

Moltke closed his eyes. 'Chancellor, since I believe it is a fact that only the beginning of a military operation is plannable, I consider it my main task to be prepared for every possible outcome of every possible situation.

Asking me if I am prepared is like asking me if I am breathing at this moment.'

'And the army?'

Moltke stiffened imperceptibly. Really, he considered such a question an insult. 'Down to the last shined boot, Chancellor.'

Thus reassured by his chief of staff, Bismarck, by various bits of skulduggery, tricked Napoleon III of France into declaring war on Prussia on 19 July 1870.

The Prussians were prepared. They mobilized immediately and drove three separate armies into France simultaneously. And Moltke guided those armies like an invisible hand.

'Preparation' wasn't in the French vocabulary at the time. They muddled through with an administration system, to which they themselves referred as 'system D for disarray'. When General Chanzy complained about lack of preparation and terrible conditions, he was told, 'Think like a Frenchman.' The implication was that French gallantry and bravery would make up for any lack of materials and preparation.

It didn't.

The French fought bravely, but the Prussians drove through them in one battle after another. Moltke, true to his word, had prepared for every possible outcome of every single engagement.

The climax came at Sedan on 1 September 1870. Napoleon III was taken prisoner, along with his entire army. Paris declared itself a commune and fought on, but the Franco-Prussian war was effectively over.

You must realize that preparation is everything – with shaving as with war.

I'm not saying that your daily shave is in the same league as the Franco-Prussian war, and I hope you don't see yourself as another Moltke. But you should prepare yourself before you place a blade on your skin. One of the most common reasons for a bad shave is insufficient preparation.

There are different ways of preparing for your shave. Most revolve around the fact that the hair on your face is tough and needs to be softened. Remember the comparison with copper wire? That's why barbers sometimes wrap a hot, wet, towel round your face.

For most of us, that isn't practical at home, unless you have someone to do it for you, so your best time to shave is after a shower, a bath, a steam bath, sauna, or whatever you've got. The theory is that the soap washes the natural oil off your stubble, allowing the water to soak in and soften it.

So, let's assume you've had your shower and now you're ready to do the deed. At this point some men shave without anything else. It's called dry-shaving. I've tried it a couple of times, but it hasn't been an enjoyable experience. Normally, we smear goo on to our faces.

Why?

- To further soften the bristles.
- To provide lubrication for the blade to glide along the skin.

LATHER

The question of what kind of goo is important. In days gone by men used goose fat, but eventually we all switched to common, everyday soap. It was in use for centuries.

Soap, incidentally, was invented by the northern Germanic tribes, and the Romans despised them for it – *they* used olive oil and scrapers to clean themselves.

Eventually common soap wasn't good enough for us any more, and we invented specialized shaving soap. This was normally sold in flakes or as a cake. A cake is still the most common way of buying it, although I remember my father rubbing shaving soap on to his cheeks from a stick, then working up a lather directly on his face with his shaving brush.

Nowadays shaving soap normally comes in a wooden bowl. You dip your brush in water, then swirl it around on the cake, adding water as you go, until the lather is the texture and consistency of beaten egg-whites.

Not content with shaving soap, we invented shaving cream, which normally comes in a tub or a tube.

The tub form is the simplest one to use. You dip your shaving brush into it, lightly since a little goes a long way, then lather it on to your face.

Shaving cream in a tube is similar. You squeeze an amount about the size of an almond into a small bowl, load your shaving brush with water, stir it in, then lather your face. Tubes are handy if you're travelling and, in general, I prefer them, these days.

Most men like to use warm or hot water to work up a lather. That makes sense from a softening and relaxing point of view. The only drawback is that hot water makes the lather on your face dry out faster than cool.

SHAVING MUGS

For the purpose of whipping up a lather, you can pilfer a mug and bowl from the kitchen, or you can buy one of those old-fashioned shaving mugs. They're a lot of fun. In case you've never seen one before, they look like the one below:

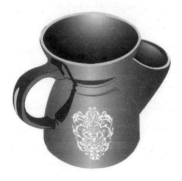

The best place to buy one is on eBay or in an antiques shop. There's a huge selection of both old and new. The prices range from next to nothing, for the plain and functional, to a small fortune for the collectable ones that are hundreds of years old.

Using them is easy: you put hot or warm water in the lower part. The large open spout is for dipping your brush in. You put the cream or soap in the top part, which normally has a couple of holes in it to let the excess water drain off, then whip up a lather.

If you're using a shaving mug with a cake of shaving soap, you have a problem: the cake will probably be a different size from the top part. How are you supposed to squeeze it in?

Don't worry. Buy whatever sized shaving soap you like, then melt it in a saucepan or microwave – be careful not to burn it – and pour it into the top part of the mug. Be sure to block off the small holes first – electrical tape on the underside works fine – or the molten soap will run into the body of the mug and you'll have a terrible time trying to get it out.

AEROSOL CANS

Men used shaving soap and brushes for a long time. Then we invented pressurized cans. Nowadays, most of the shaving cream that's sold to the men of the Western world comes in them. The good news is that they don't usually contain CFCs – chlorofluorocarbons. Originally they did, but to avoid patent restrictions the manufacturers switched to hydrocarbons – specifically, mixtures of propane, butane and isobutane – which is good news for the ozone layer.

Wait a minute! Propane? Butane? Aren't those inflammable gases? Why doesn't my head explode when I light that cigar?

Yes, hydrocarbons are highly inflammable, and butane is indeed used in cigarette lighters. But most of what's in the can is water, which is good news for cigar smokers everywhere. The bad news is the other ingredients. Recently, in the course of investigations, I went down to my local supermarket and bought at random a can of shaving foam and another of gel. Then I read the ingredients, in very fine print.

Hold on to your hats, gentlemen. Here's what's in there: aqua, palmitic acid, triethanolamine isopentane, glyceryl oleate, stearic acid, parfum, isobutane, sorbitol, hydroxyethylcellulose, ptfe, peg-90m, peg-23m, peg-150 distearate, tocopheryl acetate, propylene glycol, aloe barbadensis leaf juice, silica, bht, benzyl salicylate, butylphenyl methylpropional, hexyl cinnamal, limonene, linalool, ci42090, ci59040, propane, paraffinum liquidum, ceteareth-20, hydroxyisahexyl 3-cyclohexene carboxaldehyde.

Wow!

OK, some of the ingredients on that list are harmless. Aqua is a fancy name for water, and you can't object to that. I also happen to know that stearic acid is naturally occurring stuff – it's similar to tallow. But some of the others concerned me a little.

Triethanolamine isopentane, for example, is a solvent. It's a key component of petrol vapour. It has an anaesthetic effect on your skin, which is why they put it into shaving foam. But it can also cause breathing difficulties, dermatitis, dry skin, changing heart rhythms, headaches, dizziness and irritation in the nose and throat.

Ci42090 and ci59040 are colourings, synthetic coal-tar dyes. Ci42090 can be carcinogenic – it can give you cancer. Ci59040 is an irritant. If you splash some on your eyelids, mouth, nose or genitals, wash it off fast. The European Union forbids its use in products designed for those areas, so if you were planning on shaving down below, use something else.

Looking up this information on the web can be a lot of fun. It may also give you a heart-attack. You should read what's in your shampoo some time, or even your soap. Then sit down and wonder why roughly 30 per cent of American men will develop some form of cancer in their lifetime.

It's scandalous.

There's no reason for all of those chemicals to be packed in. If you can afford it, go upmarket: you'll find a better range of natural ingredients in your shaving cream. You're more likely, for example, to find madden root instead of Ci59040, and apricot-kernel oil instead of triethanolamine isopentane. And, trust me, those natural ingredients will make your shave a lot pleasanter.

At this point, I could include a recipe for shaving soap. I could tell you it's not that hard to make.

But I'd be lying.

Making your own shaving soap is difficult. Also, I don't believe too many men are interested in doing it. If you're seriously keen, do a web search and you'll find lots of sites that tell you how. But I believe it's beyond the scope of this book.

However, if you want to buy some really great shaving soap, do a web search using the words 'shaving soap', and 'bentonite clay' or 'fuller's clay'.

Those clays are among the best lubricants in existence. Any shaving cream that contains them is almost certainly high-quality. Several small, family-run companies make shaving soaps with such ingredients, and they're surprisingly cheap, if you consider what's in them. Here's a random sample of companies that make this kind of product. You can find them all quite easily on the web:

- Pig Dog Farm
- Daybreak Lavender Farm
- After the Rayne
- Harmony Soap Company
- Rocky Mountain Soap Company

❀ Be Good to Yourself

At this point you might be thinking, Can I justify spending so much money on myself? After all, you're probably putting all of yours into your children's college fund or your mortgage.

Right. Go into your bathroom and take a look at the storage space. If you live on your own, it's all yours. Great. But I almost guarantee that if you're living with a woman 80 per cent of the bathroom storage space is hers. I'm not arguing against that. In fact, it would be worrying if you had more space than she did. But if you only have 20 per cent of what she has, at least make certain that you fill it with good-quality products.

Of course you can justify it. And, in fact, few women would object to their men taking better care of themselves in this department since, by and large, most would like us to look and smell a little better than we currently do.

❀ Shaving Oils

If you really want to save money in this area of your life, you can use oil instead of using shaving cream. You'll find it in most supermarkets. Shaving oil is easy to use. You squeeze a little on to your fingers and rub it directly into your stubble (never use a brush with oil). Oil tends to be strong on lubrication, but the jury's out on whether it does a good job of softening your stubble.

I've tried shaving oil in the past, and it works all right, but I prefer cream.

Incidentally, other kinds of oil work all right too. I used olive oil once in a dire emergency, and it did the job. It's a handy trick to know if you run short at a crucial time in life. Be warned, though: it will leave your face smelling like something out of a Mediterranean cook-book.

SHAVING BRUSHES

You should definitely use one. Most barbers agree on this. They do a better job than you do with your fingers. There are different types on sale: synthetic, hog and badger – quite early in my shaving career, I had a brush with old badger.

THE MANY BRUSHES OF HORST

I was still a teenager, back in Germany. I had been to the Greek islands, sleeping on beaches and drinking ouzo. I was tanned, lean and broke, so I was hitchhiking home. But I stopped in Munich on the way for the Oktoberfest (which is held in September).

It was a riot. Everything revolves round drinking beer. I love beer, and I don't remember too much of anything except rivers of it, night and day, and moronic songs, which were a lot of fun.

Eventually my finances hit crisis point, and it was time to go home. But since I had pleasant memories of Munich, I took a morning to wander through the city one last time to say goodbye to places like the Marienplatz and the Augustinerhof. On the way, I came across a large department store and stepped in to look around. Actually, the main reason I stepped in was because it was raining.

In the store, I stopped at a display of shaving brushes. They looked great. I'd never seen so many on display together: they filled an enormous polished glass and mahogany case.

As I stood there, gaping, the salesman came over. I remember he was wearing a plum-coloured waistcoat with an old-fashioned tweed suit. He had a large walrus moustache and oiled hair.

'Hallo, my name is Horst.'

He spoke English to me so I must have appeared foreign. Also, he must have known that I didn't have the money to buy anything: my clothes were ragged, and I had that hungry, stony-broke look.

'You like the brushes, *ja*?'

I nodded.

'These ones here – they are all badger hair, you know.'

I nodded again, gazing at the brushes. I didn't know what to say to Horst. I thought we probably didn't have too much in common.

'And why badger, as I am sure you are asking yourself, *ja*?'

'Uuuh . . .'

'Here, I show you.'

He swung a huge set of keys out of his trouser pocket and unlocked the display case, reached in and took out a brush about the size of my fist.

'The badger, you see – his hair has the quality of water retention. The water, it soaks up. Then you dip it in the cream – the soft, luscious cream – and then you rub it on your face, very gently, like so.'

He started flicking that brush along his face in a very sensual manner.

'I tried also boar's bristle once. And, of course, young man, it is a lot better than the synthetic ones, but it does not have the qualities of the badger.'

I glanced around to see if anyone was watching. Horst swished the brush back and forth on his neck and giggled.

'The tickling is only when it is dry, you see. When it is wet, it doesn't tickle. It soothes, it massages, it anoints and makes you feel all over very wonderful.'

'Uuuh . . . I was really just looking. I'm not sure I can afford—'

Horst shook his head sadly. 'Aaah . . . money. Then I'm afraid you will have to use a synthetic brush.'

He looked at me with a glimmer of hope in his blue eyes. 'But perhaps, later in life, you will discard the synthetic brush and buy yourself one of badger. At least, I hope you will do so, young man.'

I nodded. 'Yeah, maybe. Thanks.'

Horst put the brush back into the display, and I slunk out of the shop. I forgot about badger hair for quite a while.

There are three different types of badger-hair brush:

- Pure badger: from the hair on the badger's stomach.
- Best badger: from the badger's back.
- Silvertip badger, or super-badger: from the back of the badger's neck.

I'm not denying the qualities of badger hair, and I've been reassured that most of it comes from China, where badgers are seen as a pest. But I think synthetic brushes are OK. They're cheap, and we don't have to kill helpless animals to get them.

A shaving brush should never wear out, as long as it's cared for correctly. When you finish with it, rinse it in warm water. Don't wring or squeeze it. Shake out the excess water, then hang it upside down to dry. Some men – and manufacturers – maintain that you don't need to hang it upside down. They trust to something called 'capillary action', which you should remember from your physics class at school.

But I hang mine.

So now you have your shaving cream, your brush and a bowlful of lather. Here's a tip that may be useful: no matter how fine quality your shaving brush is, soak it before you use it. Let the bristles rest for a few minutes in the warm water before you use it on your face. You'll notice a difference.

Lathering the cream on your face shouldn't be hard, but it's here that most men make their big mistake. When they've covered their faces with lather, they go straight to the shave. No. The lather needs to be worked in. Take an extra minute or two, especially on your sensitive areas, and your face will thank you for it. Don't use force: remember, only the tips of the hairs produce the lather, so be gentle with that brush. Some men like to add more water at this point, for a really wet shave, but you can stick with the egg-white consistency. It all depends on your personal preference. The important point is not to rush the lathering.

SUMMARY CHECKLIST

- ✢ For your next birthday, when your mum or live-in lover asks you what you want, ask them to buy you a shaving brush, and use it well.

- ✢ Be good to yourself: buy the most expensive shaving cream you can afford.

- ✢ Lather, lather, lather: you can never have too much of a good thing.

- ✢ Read *Wind in the Willows* a few times, then buy a synthetic brush.

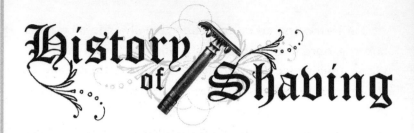

History of Shaving

THE ROMANS

Initially the Romans were bearded, but shaving crept in from the Greek colonies in southern Italy. General Scipio Africanus was the first major figure to shave daily. But it was Julius Caesar — he was naturally bald — who popularized the clean-shaven look. Julius didn't shave, though: he preferred his facial hair to be pulled out with tweezers.

After Caesar, the pattern was set. Romans shaved for centuries, and the rich and powerful wouldn't be seen dead in public with stubble. It was a manly duty that they took seriously.

The rich had their own barbers on their household staff; the rest of the population went to public institutions, of which there were two types:

- The more expensive, indoor variety (*tonstrinae*), which had polished mirrors on the walls, and benches where you could wait and discuss state affairs with your peers.

- The downmarket, open-air variety, where you sat on the ground to wait, and where any distracting incident in the street might cause your barber to do you a serious injury.

The Etruscans – just before the Romans – used bronze razors, with three-holed grips for your fingers. But we have no idea what Roman razors (*novacila*) looked like: they were made of iron, which has not survived the passage of time. We do know, however, that they could not make tempered steel so the razors were blunt. Also, they had only polished metal as mirrors and no shaving soap.

In a word, shaving was hell. As Martial wrote,

These scars on my chin, if you can count them, may look like those on a boxer's face, but they were not caused that way, nor by the sharp talons of a fierce wife, but by the accursed steel and hand of the barber Antiochus.

After the barber had finished with you, though, he would patch up the mess he had made of your face by applying a soothing plaster made of perfumed ointments and spider webs soaked in oil and vinegar. And if you lost your nerve and chose a depilatory cream instead of a blade, things weren't much better. Among other ingredients, it might have contained resin, pitch, goats' gall, bats' blood and powdered viper.

Roman shaving habits, along with hairstyles, were largely

determined by the emperor of the day. The Emperor Marcus Aurelius took it all one step further, shaving his entire head. But then the Emperor Hadrian – the man who built the wall across northern England – had warts and battle-scars on his face, so he grew a beard to cover them. That meant beards were back in fashion until Constantine the Great, the first Christian Emperor, came down against them.

Shaving off your first facial growth was an important rite of passage into manhood for the Romans. Friends and family gathered for the celebration, and the hair from the first shave was preserved in a box and sacrificed to one of the gods. In the case of the emperors Nero and Caligula, their first shave happened at the same time as their donning of the toga: the official, legal coming-of-age ceremony. Nero sacrificed his hair to Jupiter Capitoline in a gold box.

Much as today, Roman youth would sometimes not shave in order to draw a reaction from their elders. Even then stubble was a form of protest.

Finally, spare a thought for the Roman legions, stationed in some godforsaken wilderness crawling with barbarians. They had neither the time nor the barbers for shaving, so they used pumice stones to rub off their facial hair. This method had the advantage of practicality.

The disadvantage? Well, try rubbing off your stubble with a pumice stone some day.

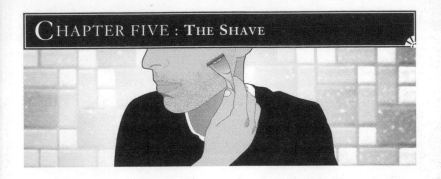

When I was younger and didn't know much about anything, my karate teacher stopped me once in mid-fight: 'You're too tense,' he said. 'You must train hard, but fight easy.'

I didn't understand what he meant, but he knocked it into my thick head until the principle sank in. You put in all the hard work before the actual performance. When you're performing the task for which you've trained, you shouldn't be tense. If your body and mind are prepared, you should relax into total self-confidence when fighting. This is what I understand from these lines:

> In the void is virtue, and no evil. Wisdom
> has existence, principle has existence, the
> way has existence, spirit is nothingness.

A modern volleyball coach might put it like this: 'You're in the zone. You can't miss. Every move feels right. Every touch on the ball feels perfect.'

Most athletes have experienced that sensation at some point. And they know that you only enter the zone after a lot of hard training.

Shaving is the same. If you've done your preparation well, you'll probably have a good shave. So, now is the time to release the tension. Don't grip your blade as if it were a shovel. Hold it easy and relaxed and, while you're at it, relax the rest of yourself. I like listening to Pink Floyd while I'm shaving.

Before we move on to shaving technique, though, we must study two important points:

- The grain of your beard.
- Stretching your skin.

THE GRAIN OF YOUR BEARD

People's facial hair grows in different directions. Mostly, on the cheeks, it grows downwards. But on the neck and chin areas everyone's different. You need to find out and understand which way yours grows.

At a time when your stubble is short, normally about twenty-four hours after your last shave, run your fingers over it, in different directions. When you go in one direction, you'll feel resistance. When you go in the opposite direction, it will feel almost smooth, as if you don't need a shave. The direction that feels smooth is the one in which the hair is growing.

It's important to know this, and it's connected to a fundamental question: should you shave with or against the grain? Everyone has a different opinion on this one, even professional barbers.

My opinion is this: in all cases, the first pass the blade makes over your face should be *with* the grain. It's painful to go against the grain on the first pass, and you stand a higher risk of nicking yourself.

When you've finished the first pass, you can, if you wish, take a second pass. This pass should be at a ninety-degree angle *across* the grain.

If you wish, you can take a third pass, *against* the grain.

So, for example, if we assume that the grain of your beard is downwards on your cheeks – as it is with most men – you would shave your cheeks first from your ear to your jawline, then across, from your eye towards your ear, then upwards, from your jawline towards your ear.

Taking three passes has its advantages: you achieve the ultimate close shave, which can be important if you're planning on getting close to someone. The problem is that you're also slicing off a fair amount of epidermis. It all depends on how sensitive your skin is. If you're experiencing discomfort, stick with one pass. I take a second pass across my cheeks, but leave the rest of my face on just one. That gets me plenty close enough.

If you're going to take more than one pass, I recommend

you lather again between passes, although this can be time-consuming. If a barber shaves you, he'll normally take at least a second pass. If you don't want that, tell him to stick with one. A good barber should know what you're talking about.

The question of how many passes, with or against the grain, is something you should consider. Shaving should be enjoyable. If you're hurting yourself, it normally means you're going too close, which in turn means that either you're going against – or across – the grain, or that you're taking too many passes.

I have a concern in this matter regarding the multi-bladed disposables. If you're using a cut-throat razor, or a single-blade disposable, and take three separate passes, you've passed the blade over your skin three times. But if you take three separate passes with a five-bladed razor, you're actually passing fifteen blades across your cheeks. And if you take multiple strokes for one pass, your skin could have upwards of twenty to thirty blades going over it, which may lead to irritation and razor-burn.

Everyone has his own preference. But if I had to give advice on this one, I'd say 'Be kind to your face.' Shaving is primarily a visual thing. No one will notice if you haven't gone right down. They will, however, notice if you've gone down too deep. Razor-burn is noticeable, even from a distance. Also, you'll do your face no good in the long term by going too close.

THE BUSINESS MEETING

Once I had to attend a business meeting where I was out of my depth. I had a shave and put on a suit. I hate wearing a suit at the best of times, and that day was among the worst because it was sweltering hot. I felt as if my tie was throttling me, and I wished that I could be anywhere but where I was.

Then my counterpart on the other side turned up, and I suddenly felt much more relaxed. He had shaved himself far too close. There were red patches of razor-burn on his neck and round his mouth. I spotted at least two nicks. He had also splashed on a bucketful of alcohol-based aftershave, which filled the room with its stink. It made him itch. Beads of sweat ran down his cheeks, and he kept rubbing and scratching at his face. He might as well have screamed his insecurity from the rooftops, and even though he was on the other side, I felt sorry for him.

STRETCHING YOUR SKIN

Most men understand this instinctively: your skin needs to be taut when you shave it. This leads us into various contortions: jutting our chins, craning our necks, rolling our eyeballs up at the ceiling. It makes us look ridiculous, but there's no way round it. Keeping your skin taut is crucial: if it's loose, the blade (or blades) will push a mound of skin in front of it, then slice into that mound. That's how you nick yourself.

Don't be tempted to pull the skin too taut, though, since that can have adverse effects too, like razor-burn. In general, it should never feel uncomfortable.

❋ SHAVING THE CHEEKS

In theory, you can start the shave wherever you want. In reality, most men start at their sideburns and shave their cheeks, so that's where we'll start too. Your cheeks are the easiest area of your face to shave since, normally, they're a large flat surface.

Dig your fingers into your sideburns and stretch the skin upwards. Place the blade, whether it's a cut-throat or a safety, at roughly a thirty-degree angle to your skin and pull the blade down towards your jawline.

That thirty-degree angle is important to bear in mind. The advantage of a safety razor is that, on most of them, the head has been angled like this already. With a cut-throat, you need to replicate that angle. For some reason, a lot of men switch to a very steep angle when they start to use a cut-throat. You can increase the angle *a little* with a cut-throat, until you become used to it. But you cannot place the blade at a ninety-degree angle to your skin and try to scrape away the stubble. Remember that you're cutting the hair exactly as you would with a safety razor.

If you're using a cut-throat, you probably only need to

go over your cheeks once or twice. If it's a safety, you might need to repeat the strokes several times. Use whatever pressure feels good to you, but remember to hold the skin taut.

When your safety razor is clogged with lather, rinse it, either under a running tap, or by swirling it around in the wash-basin. Here's where I have my biggest problem with the multi-bladed safety razor: you have to keep rinsing until all the hairs are cleared, which takes time. You don't rinse a cut-throat at all: you wipe it clean on a piece of paper. And you can easily shave half of your face without wiping the blade. It doesn't clog.

When you've finished your cheeks, you normally move on to your chin or neck. It doesn't matter which you do first. Perceived wisdom is that you should leave your chin until last, since the bristles are toughest there, but it's a matter of personal choice.

SHAVING THE CHIN

When you do your chin, keep the skin taut. Most men grip one side of their skin to stretch it. Try stretching it from both sides, with your middle finger and thumb, as shown on p. 100.

It will feel more comfortable, especially if you have a cleft or dimpled chin, like Kirk Douglas or Rock Hudson. The only way to shave that bit is to stretch it.

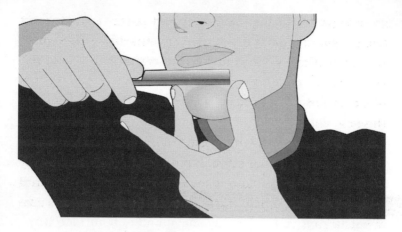

Incidentally, many men's chin hair grows straight out – there is, therefore, no 'grain'. So it doesn't matter if you go from left to right or vice versa. Go with whatever direction feels comfortable.

SHAVING THE NECK

On your neck there is most definitely a grain – or, rather, two grains. The stubble there normally shows a dividing line where it switches the direction of its growth. Some men also have whorls where it grows in every direction. This is a recipe for trouble.

When shaving the neck, try to go with the grain as far as possible. I recommend this even if you're taking a second or third pass. Also, there's nothing wrong with lathering a second or third time if you feel you need to.

I see a lot of men with tiny red spots on their neck from shaving. This is mostly because they've gone against the grain or taken too many passes. If that's the case with you, stick to one pass and take time to work out the different grains on your neck. This knowledge will pay off in the long run.

While I'm on the subject of the neck, directly under the jawline is another difficult bit for many men. The only trick I can give you here is to pull the skin upwards until it's right over your jaw, so that you shave that area as part of your cheeks.

SHAVING AROUND THE MOUTH

Most men leave this area and their upper lip to last. It can be tough, and the upper lip may be sensitive, which is why many men grow moustaches. That's an important point to bear in mind: some men's moustaches and goatees are not fashion statements – they simply find this area difficult to shave and take the logical way out. Think about the moustaches of Adolf Hitler and Charlie Chaplin, then consider this: I know several men whose eyes water when they shave directly under their nose, no matter how careful they are. In fact, now I come to think of it, mine did when I started shaving, but as my technique improved and my blade grew sharper, it stopped.

Most men's upper-lip hair grows directly down, not

So, you've finished your shave. Now rinse your face thoroughly with warm water to remove the last remnants of lather. Then rinse it with cold water (skip this part if it's mid-winter and you're not feeling up to it). The theory behind the hot/cold thing is that the warm water opens the pores and allows everything to be washed away, the cold water closes them again. Cold water is also refreshing, which may be important if you put too much beer or Scotch into yourself the night before.

When you've finished rinsing, you may notice that a trickle of blood is leaking out here and there. If you've made a really bad job of it, it may be flowing in a steady stream. But even if you've only scraped yourself, or if your skin is feeling a bit tender, you may find yourself asking: 'Why do men have to do this?'

We Do This Because We Are Men

In the course of my life I've studied many medieval manuscripts. I've spent several years immersed in restricted sections of dusty libraries, reading ancient lapidaries or herbariums that, even in their day, never made it on to any bestseller list. But every so often I stumbled across something great. One such text concerned the ill-fated French crusade, which ran from 1249 to 1250. Even though they were on a mission to liberate the holy city of Jerusalem, the French crusaders ended up in Egypt.

Things didn't work out so great for them, and they went through their fair share of suffering. Here's a contemporary account by the chronicler Jean de Joinville of the after-effects of one particular battle:

> Sir Hugues d'Escosse was desperately hurt by three great wounds in the face and elsewhere. Sir Raoul and Sir Ferreys were also badly wounded in their shoulders, so that the blood spouted out just like to a tun of wine when tapped. Sir Errart d'Esmeray was so severely wounded in the face by a sword, the stroke of which cut off his nose, that it hung down over his mouth.

Despite their wounds, they all fought on. I like that.

Shaving discomfort isn't in the same league as the French crusade. Nevertheless, there are some steps you should consider if your shave doesn't feel good:

- Reduce the number of passes you take to one or two instead of three. Go with the grain instead of against it.
- Give your face a rest. Shaving is an efficient way of exfoliating your skin, and women nowadays pay a lot of money for exfoliation creams. But would a woman exfoliate every day? No chance. Let your stubble grow

at least one day a week. If you're dark-haired, this might have to be over the weekend. If you're fair-haired, you can skip your shave any day you like. Your face will thank you for it and your boss won't notice.

- Use a sharp razor: blunt and worn blades play hell with your skin. If you're using a cut-throat razor, maintain it well (see Chapter 7). If you employ a safety razor, don't use it for months on end, as I once did.

- Don't rush your shave: you'll do a sloppy job. If you don't have time to shave, don't shave. The world won't come to an end because you skipped one, and it doesn't mean you're a degenerate Communist.

- If the area round your mouth is tender and you find it impossible to do a decent job there, consider one of two things: buy yourself a single-blade disposable for that bit, saving the multi-blade one for your cheeks and neck. Alternatively, grow a goatee. See how you like it.

If you've ignored all the advice in this chapter, and, consequently, you're bleeding now, with raw, tenderized skin, rest assured: the next chapter deals with mopping-up operations. Please try not to bleed on the book.

Summary Checklist

✦ Understand which way the grain on your face lies.

✦ Be kind to your face. Shave with the grain, at least on the first pass.

✦ Keep your blade sharp.

✦ Keep your skin taut, but not too taut.

✦ Keep that thirty-degree angle constant.

✦ Be glad you weren't a crusader.

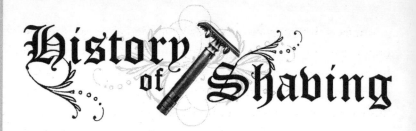

History of Shaving

THE MIDDLE AGES AND BEYOND

In the middle ages, fashions changed from time to time and from locality to locality. William the Conqueror was dead against facial hair, and after he took England, he made the local Saxons cut off their flowing moustaches. Many emigrated, rather than contemplate life without their essential badge of manhood.

Ivan the Terrible, Tsar of Russia and possibly the most mentally unstable ruler since Caligula, held with beards in a big way, and if you shaved yours off, you could be thrown to a pack of half-starved hunting dogs, with Ivan cheering them on. When Elizabeth I of England sent her ambassadors to visit him, one had such long moustaches that Ivan came down from his throne to play with them.

When Peter the Great became tsar, he decided that beards were archaic and taxed anyone who wore one. To reinforce the point, he took to shaving off his nobles' beards himself, in public, and he didn't have a gentle touch. The peasants, of course, were exempt from this tax, as long as they kept ploughing.

In fact, the toing and froing with shaving affected only the upper classes. Your average peasant ploughed and toiled with his beard intact. Nothing fazed him. The peasant is like some great shaggy dog running through history, unwashed and unshaven. For some reason I find that comforting.

The men who suffered most from these vicissitudes were the barbers. Their career fluctuated with the times, and perhaps because of this they decided to diversify in a bizarre way. They took up surgery and dentistry on the side.

Here's how that came about.

When the Roman Empire collapsed, Europe descended into an age of darkness. It's a good lesson in what happens when warriors take control. Everyone forgot how to read and write. Nobody washed. Even those at the top of the food chain – the lords – were illiterate and stinking. What was important was that you knew how to handle your sword. Otherwise your life was, quite literally, cut short.

In this kind of environment people were hurt a lot, and when they were hurt they went to a physician. The best physicians were the monks and priests, since they were the only ones who remembered how to read and write. When they needed an assistant with a sharp blade – to do some bloodletting, for example – they sent for the local barber. It was a question of convenience: barbers were best able to use a sharp blade delicately and with precision.

In 1163, though, the Catholic Church held the Council of Tours at which Pope Alexander III decreed that the clergy were forbidden to draw blood from the human body: it was sacrilegious. After that, the barbers took over the whole show. Your local barber became your local surgeon. And they didn't stick with bloodletting: they went in for other operations too, most notably amputation. From major surgery it was only a short jump to dentistry. After all, for that they needed only a pair of pliers and a strong wrist.

The red-and-white-striped pole originated in those dark times. Barbers started using it for two reasons:

- To give the patient something to grip as the blade (or saw, in the case of an amputation) went in. Anaesthetics didn't exist back then.

- To dry the bloodied bandages. They would hang them from the pole, then put it outside. The wind wrapped the bandages round the pole, in a pattern of red and white stripes.

After a while, the poles became symbolic, the stripes painted on, the same poles you see outside barber shops today.

Not surprisingly, barbers earned themselves a grisly reputation. Standards were abysmal, and they killed many of their patients. Sometimes people only had to see them coming to drag themselves out of bed and run for it.

In response to this state of affairs, the brotherhoods of St Cosmos and St Domain were formed in Paris in the thirteenth century. In London, the Worshipful Company of

Barbers – still in existence today – was founded. These institutions became the most advanced medical training schools of the age. They tied in with the guilds of barbers and surgeons, which were responsible for maintaining standards and controlling the industry.

Gradually, thank goodness, the surgeons gained the upper hand and broke away from the barbers. In the fifteenth century barbers were restricted to pulling teeth, bloodletting and cauterization. They weren't allowed to cut off your legs any more. It was the beginning of the end, but it was only in 1745 that in England an Act of Parliament ensured that the two professions finally went their separate ways.

From the late seventeenth century shaving technology improved in leaps and bounds. The first recognizable cut-throat razor appeared in Sheffield in 1680, and by the middle of the eighteenth century, excellent-quality blades were available. Shaving soap had been invented, and people were starting to use aftershave, notably cherry laurel water in the Victorian age. Also, the shaving brush had come into its own, reducing the phenomenon known as 'barber's itch', caused by filthy sponges or fingers used to create a lather.

Gradually the local barbershop ceased to be a place of pain and became instead a pleasant all-male environment where you went for a daily penny shave and the latest gossip. It was where you met your fellow men and talked, or listened, where decisions were taken, stories told and male wisdom passed on.

CHAPTER SIX : MOPPING UP

When people hear that I use a cut-throat razor, they always ask the same question: 'Do you cut yourself often?'

I laugh. No, as a rule, I don't. Of course, I might behead the odd pimple, like the rest of the male population, but I don't cut myself. Why would I?

THE CHINESE OPIUM DEN ❋

Except I did, a few years ago.

It was the office Christmas party, and there was a wide selection of single-malt Scotch behind the bar. There were Cuban cigars too, which we could put on the tab. Everything got a little out of control, and when I made it home, at about four in the morning, I barely managed to crawl up the stairs on all fours. Everything was spinning.

In a spiritual epiphany, I decided to have a shave.

The lathering part went fine, and I stropped the blade

fairly well, but as the steel touched my cheekbone, I hesitated, and blinked. What was I doing?

When I pulled away the razor, a line of deepest red appeared across my cheek. I had enough presence of mind to put away the blade safely (I have young children) and crawled into bed. I didn't use a styptic. In fact, I fell asleep with my face still lathered.

The next morning, I wasn't a pleasant sight. I had to go to work, and the cut was spectacular. It was at least three inches across – disposable razorblades aren't made that wide. I was working for a well-known multinational company, and I was supposed to be well groomed at all times.

To everyone who asked at work – and they all did – I told the truth: I'd cut myself shaving.

No one believed me: they all wanted to hear a story of a terrific knife-fight in a pub. After a while, I couldn't help myself. It was over lunch. My colleagues and managers were all there, and every so often one would look in my direction, shake his head knowingly and smile. They were wondering what I'd been hit with: a bottle, a knife, an enraged woman's claws?

My manager grinned at me. 'Come on, tell us what really happened. We're dying to know.'

I put down my spoon. 'OK, I didn't cut myself shaving.'

They leaned closer.

'No. After I left you, I took myself off to this opium den I go to sometimes.'

My manager's eyes popped.

'So there I was, with my bamboo pipe, sucking in the sweet black smoke, with a naked Chinese lady beside me, and this brilliant opium wave washing over me, and I'm about to go off to the misty lands where reality has no meaning . . .'

Everyone was listening now.

'. . . when this crazy man bursts in and whacks me across the side of the head with a machcte.'

I picked up my spoon and got on with my soup.

They were gaping at me.

'Really?'

I closed my eyes. 'To tell the truth, I can't remember. But it's either that or I cut myself shaving.'

STYPTICS

No matter how good you are, you will cut yourself sometimes, or behead a pimple. When this happens, the answer is not to press a damp wad of toilet paper on to your face. The answer is a styptic.

A styptic stops the flow of blood by sealing the cut. It comes in three forms:

- A styptic pencil – the most common type. It looks like a stick of lip-balm. It's normally white. Application is quite easy: you rub it on where it's needed. If you do

it straight away, no one need know that you cut
yourself.

- A styptic powder. Exactly the same principle as a
styptic pencil, except that it's a bit messier to apply;
you use a cotton-wool bud, such as Q-tips.
- A block of alum. My perennial favourite, for various
reasons. Alum is a double sulphate of alumina and
potash, which means it's a mineral salt. You buy it in
a block that looks like a cake of soap or maybe a lump
of cracked ice. It's hard to describe. Buy one and you'll
see.

Alum is a good styptic, but sometimes I use it as
an aftershave, rubbing it over my whole face. I like
it because it makes my skin feel taut and smooth
as hell. And when I use it like that, it serves as a
good yardstick.

Yardstick?

Listen, try this: after you've finished your shave, leave
your face wet. Run the alum under the cold tap, then rub
it gently over your face. Don't go too close to your lips
since alum doesn't taste great.

When you rub it on, you'll probably find that it tingles
a lot in some areas, and less so in others. If that's the case
(and almost certainly it will be) you're giving yourself an
uneven shave.

Look on that as a challenge. You should be shaving
yourself with the same closeness all over your face.
Adjust. Rectify it. Become a better shaver. That's what I

mean by 'yardstick'. I'm continually trying to improve my shaving technique, and you should too.

You can buy a styptic pencil in any decent men's razor-supplies shop, and on the Internet. Alum is harder to come by. The Internet might be your best bet. Use a search engine. To give yourself a wider choice of web-sites, be aware that several companies sell it under its French name: 'bloc Osma'.

A word of warning on styptics though: you shouldn't share your pencil, for obvious health reasons. And if you're in a barbershop, he nicks you and reaches for the styptic pencil, I recommend you say, 'No.' If your barber knows his business, he won't nick you. But if by any chance he does, he should be using powdered styptic, with a disposable cotton-wool bud. That way you won't pick up an infection.

Finally, as with most mineral salts, be aware that alum can be seriously corrosive to metal, so if you get it on your razor, you should wash it off before you put it away.

AFTERSHAVE LOTION

After the styptic, it's time to think about some kind of aftershave. Let's start off with alcohol-based aftershave lotions, which is what most men in the Western world splash on.

When aftershave lotion entered the public consciousness, especially in America, real men weren't supposed to wear it. It was only for sissies or pansies. Before the First World War, you might smell witch hazel or bay rum on a man, but that was the full extent of it. Really dashing men might put a dab of their wife's perfume under their jacket lapel.

Then along came an Italian actor.

VALENTINO

It's hard to understand now what all the fuss was about. Lots of people have never heard of Rudolph Valentino or, if they have, only in the context of a joke – as a kind of Casanova figure.

But back in the 1920s Valentino was very real indeed. He was one of the most accomplished screen lovers of all time. His finest hour came in *The Sheikh*, in which he had several romantic scenes with one Agnes Ayres, where he was alternately cruel and violent, tender and caring. Nowadays the scenes may seem a little tame, but back then they were sensational. Women fainted in the aisles. Newspapers ran editorials. Something approaching mass *Sheikh* hysteria swept America. People decorated their living rooms to look like Bedouin tents. Lots of younger men wanted to be like Valentino, but the more traditional type were outraged: this pampered, preening Italian sissy was leading the young astray from the true path of masculinity.

Valentino used a heavy, citrus-based cologne that

filled a room with its scent. This was something new for women, and they reacted enthusiastically. Valentino didn't try to dampen things down: he had numerous affairs with both men and women. For a while he worked as a gigolo and married the bisexual girlfriend of one of his leading ladies. That didn't work out, so he married again, but without being divorced first, and was thrown into jail for bigamy. Eventually he ended up with Pola Negri, a sultry actress who would turn up at parties with a pet panther on a leash.

Valentino was a clean-shaven man. In fact, when he cultivated a beard for *The Hooded Falcon*, the barbers of America vowed to boycott his films until he shaved it off. In the midst of a media circus, Valentino bowed to the pressure and shaved.

In the end, while he was touring the country to promote his final film, the *Chicago Times* ran an editorial accusing him of the 'effeminization of the American male'. Valentino demanded a boxing match with the journalist.

Wisely, the journalist preferred to remain anonymous, so Valentino climbed into the ring with a sports writer, Frank O'Neil. He floored O'Neil with two straight punches, then went on to an all-night party. After the party, he collapsed in agony in his room. He was rushed to hospital, but fell into a coma and died. The official cause of death was peritonitis caused by a ruptured appendix and perforated ulcers.

His funeral was quite a spectacle. The police lost control of the crowd of mourning women, who stormed the funeral parlour, breaking through the glass window. Many were injured in the ensuing stampede. Quite a few of his more dedicated fans committed suicide. After Valentino the world of the American male would never be the same.

Aftershave and cologne were here to stay, and today most men wear it, without fear of being called sissy, pansy or worse.

So, what does aftershave do?

I'm going to get a little technical here, but not too much so because – I admit it – chemistry always confused the hell out of me. But bear with me on the two points below:

- Your skin has a chemical barrier called the 'stratum corneum'. It's there to prevent water escaping, and bacteria entering.
- Many aftershave lotions contain alcohol, and also something called monoterpenes.

Monoterpenes dissolve the fatty parts of the stratum corneum, so the alcohol will penetrate to your pain receptors very easily indeed. It excites them.

YOW!

Alcohol-based aftershave stings.

In fact, if you've done a good enough job of tenderizing your skin while shaving, it will feel like the napalm of my very first shave.

The flip side of that pain is that it lasts only a few seconds. But in those seconds, the pain triggers a release of endorphins in the brain, which produces an effect similar to a drug-induced high. That's what accounts for the 'bracing' effect.

What that means in non-technical terms is, yes, it stings, but a lot of men like the feeling. If you're one of them, you might as well run with it. It's your life.

Apart from the 'bracing' sensation, most men use it because it's perfumed. That's right, there's perfume in it. Men wear it for the same reason women do. Ask any teenage boy who's splashed on some of his dad's Old Spice. It's a question of smelling good for the girls to make them more friendly.

THE MONKS' DISCO

My first experience with aftershave lotion actually predates my first shave by a good few years – probably like most teenagers'.

I was in Switzerland, high in the mountains, in an old monastery boarding-school run by Benedictine monks. It was very strange. I used to be an altar-boy, but that doesn't come into this story.

The boarders were all boys. There were a few girls in the school, but they were day pupils so we didn't see much of them. Anyway, there weren't enough to go round. Competition was tough.

But, by and large, those Benedictine monks were a

liberal bunch. They let us hold a school disco about once a year. And, as anyone who's been to a school disco knows, those events give rise to expectations in teenage boys. We were no exception. We cleaned up. I put on my coolest clothes and slicked back my hair. Picture John Travolta in *Grease* and you'll have the general idea.

I wasn't old enough to shave. None of us was, thank God. That humiliation came years later. But one boy in the class had something special: Russian Leather after-shave lotion. It came in a white plastic bottle. The smell was masculine. How did we know it was masculine? Because it said so on the bottle.

The problem was, the boy who owned the bottle – let's call him Stefan – wasn't a friend. He could conjugate Latin verbs correctly, which meant that either he wasn't in my gang or I wasn't in his. And because of this, he decided to harm my chances with the girls. The swine wouldn't share his Russian Leather. In fact, he wouldn't give anyone so much as a dab, although we tried hard to persuade him . . .

'Let me have just a little, Stefan. I only want to see if it smells OK.'

'Go and buy your own.'

'Don't be such a hog.'

'You're not old enough to wear aftershave.'

'I'm two months older than you.'

'But mentally you're years younger. You have to be

mature to wear Russian Leather. It's an aftershave for men, not boys.'

'Swine.'

'Now I definitely won't give you any.'

We went on and on, but we couldn't persuade him. In the end he left us with no choice but to steal it. As soon as he had gone to the disco with his friends, we ransacked his wardrobe and found it stashed cunningly among his socks.

We musked-up with intent. We weren't given to compromise. Between seven of us, we emptied the bottle. My eyes watered with the fumes.

Then we ran off to the disco, where we danced a lot. And as we worked up a sweat we made that dance hall reek of Russian Leather. People complained of the stench, but we didn't care. That was the start of my glory years on the dance floor.

Throughout my teenage and early shaving years, I used cheap, alcohol-based aftershave lotions. Every disco I went to, I splashed it on liberally. My definition of enough was when my eyes watered. Now I can't honestly say whether the girls liked it. I probably stank like a rutting wildebeest, but I didn't care. I had my fair share of success, so I suppose they can't have minded too much. Then again, a lot of the girls smelt just as strongly of cheap perfume.

AFTERSHAVE BALM

In addition to stinging your face, alcohol-based aftershave lotions may irritate and dry your skin. When this became generally known in the Western world, manufacturers came up with aftershave balm. This is normally a cream that's marketed as being kind to your face, as well as non-stinging. The non-stinging part is generally true, but be careful: some – especially the scented ones – still contain alcohol. If you really want to go down the health track, you can just slap aloe vera gel on your face. Aloe vera is a great moisturizer, and it doesn't contain any of those frightening-sounding chemicals that you find in other aftershave products.

My experience with balm started when I was eighteen. I hitchhiked to Munich in my summer holidays and worked on the production line at BMW. I earned a lot of money and had a whale of a time – so much so, in fact, that at the end of the summer I was stony broke and had to hitchhike home again. I didn't have the money for a train ticket.

But one of the things I brought home with me was a bottle of very expensive aftershave balm.

It was great. That is, it smelt great. On one occasion, in fact, its scent was solely responsible for an unexpected success I had with a girl. She told me so. She didn't like me – she just wanted more of the smell.

TALC AND ALUM

But the balm made my skin a bit greasy so I switched again. This happened after my first cut-throat razor shave in a barbershop in Abu Dhabi.

After the shave, the barber dried my face thoroughly, then dusted it off with a brush dipped in talc. It felt great: silky, smooth and dry. I went straight out and bought myself a bottle of finely ground, sandalwood-scented talc. I used talc for several years afterwards. One of the good things about it is that a bottle lasts nearly for ever. I could use it on my sweaty feet and under my armpits too.

Then I discovered alum and used that for several years.

Incidentally, alum is in widespread use as an after-shave in India, but practically nowhere else. And although talc is widely used in the Arab world, I don't know anyone who uses it in the West. It seems to be a case of different aftershave products for different cultures.

The disadvantage of alum – or advantage for some men – is that it has no scent. That's not really a problem, though: if you want to smell nice, splash cologne on your chest, or bite the bullet and buy yourself some men's perfume. They sell it now and attitudes are changing. Blame Valentino.

❄ Skin Food

Finally, quite recently, I bought a bottle of lime-scented aftershave skin food from Geo F. Trumper's.

Trumper's is a great barbershop in London, an institution, really. Its history goes back to the glory days of the British Empire, and the company makes its own line of shaving products. I stop off there to pick up a few things when I'm in London, and I'm never disappointed. The shop itself is a work of art: all dark wood and display cases, with polished glass and coloured liquids. It reminds me of a medieval alchemist's laboratory.

Trumper's skin food is a bit more liquid than most aftershave balms but you massage it in in exactly the same way. It smells nice, and it doesn't leave your skin feeling greasy. It's also supposed to be a healthy option, but I'm not going to endorse that until I've used it for a few years.

Nowadays, I alternate between alum and skin food, depending on what mood I'm in. I don't use talc or alcohol-based aftershaves at all, unless I feel like taking a trip down Memory Lane. And I never wore Russian Leather after that first disco: some memories are sacred.

Most men try a couple of different aftershaves when they're teenagers and stick with one for upwards of thirty years. You should experiment with a range of products before you settle on one. Obviously, if you have a very positive or negative reaction to any of the above, you should take it into consideration. People with allergies must be especially careful.

SCENT

Alcohol-based aftershaves offer the widest selection of scents. The only one I'll mention here, though, is Dominica Bay Rum. It has its own distinctive smell and a long history. It was first made in the West Indies: the leaves of the bay tree were boiled in white rum and the distilled vapours collected. It contains bay oil, citrus, spice oils, alcohol and water. It made its way into the North American consciousness via the California Antilles Trading Consortium – still in operation today. You'll either love it or hate it. There's no middle ground. I think it makes you smell like a pirate, which I suppose can be a good or a bad thing, depending on how you feel about pirates.

While I'm on the subject of scent, if you're single you should go with the one that suits you. If you're in a steady relationship, I recommend a test-run with your better half. Take them to the shop with you. If you choose the wrong one – one that they find nauseating – be prepared for a significant drop in closeness. Scent is practically the number-one factor in the laws of attraction. It's probably been responsible for the dumping of a lot of men, who are left to wonder what they've done wrong.

Summary Checklist

+ Buy a styptic pencil.

+ Buy a block of alum.

+ Buy some talc, aftershave balm and skin food. Try them all out and settle on the one you prefer.

+ Never shave while drunk.

+ Teenage boys, go easy on the aftershave.

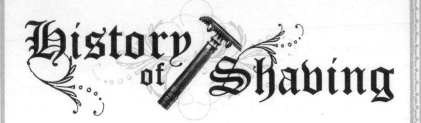

History of Shaving

THE DEMON BARBER OF FLEET STREET

I need to make something clear: I like barbers. Really, I've never met one who wasn't friendly. That's why writing about Sweeney Todd is tough for me. But there's a dark side to the history of shaving, and his story has to be told. No book on shaving would be complete without it. If you're squeamish, you can skip this chapter. I won't be offended.

Sweeney Todd lived in eighteenth-century England. Times were hard. The Industrial Revolution was in full swing, and no one really understood how to handle it. Factories demanded labour, and large numbers of people moved around the place, which caused problems. People starved and died of various sicknesses. Many froze to death, and a fair few were murdered. Crime was out of control. There was no organized police force. There were a few sheriffs and local magistrates, but not nearly enough to cope.

And then there was gin.

The lower classes took to gin in a big way. In one year, England drank eight million gallons. That caused social problems, with babies being left in the streets to die and people stabbing each other in public.

The black spot of the nation was London. Its slums were terrifying, but the poor and dispossessed flocked there from all corners of England. There was next to no law, and only a bare semblance of order.

Sweeney Todd was born in London, where his parents worked in a silk factory. One night, when he was twelve, they left him alone and went off to find some gin, even though it was one of the coldest winters London had ever experienced. They found their gin, drank it and went to sleep on the street, where they froze solid.

Sweeney Todd was now an orphan, and the parish had to take care of him, which in due course it did: it apprenticed him.

We don't really have an apprenticeship system any more – at least, not in the way it existed back then. And that's a good thing because, in effect, an apprenticeship was a kind of fixed-term slavery. You more or less belonged to your master, and what he ordered you to do, you did.

Sweeney Todd was apprenticed to a cutler, a highly skilled professional who made, repaired and sharpened knives, scissors and cut-throat razors. As such, Sweeney Todd became an expert in making and sharpening blades. But since his master was also a thief, it meant he became one, too, and he wasn't very good at that. When he was fourteen, he was caught, and came close to being hanged — in those days children were hanged for stealing handkerchiefs. Unusually, the judge took pity on him because he was an orphan and sentenced him instead to five years in prison.

Those five years were formative ones for the young Sweeney Todd. In prison, he became a kind of informal apprentice to the prison barber, shaving the prisoners before they were hanged, so when he walked out, a free man at the age of nineteen, he had a trade. He worked as a 'flying barber', which meant he didn't have a shop and plied his trade where he could. At this point in his life, he almost certainly committed the odd murder with robbery, and a few years later he had enough money to set himself up with premises on Fleet Street, where he hung up his sign:

Easy shaving for a penny
As good as you will find any.

There, he cut his customers' hair, shaved them and sometimes pulled out their teeth. And when the mood caught him, he'd murder one.

It happened like this.

The customer would sit back in the barber's chair, ready for his shave. Sweeney Todd would pull a lever that opened a trapdoor. The chair would swing backwards and the customer would fall quite a distance into a deep basement. The clever part of the arrangement was that a second barber's chair would swing up to replace the first. The picture should give you the general idea:

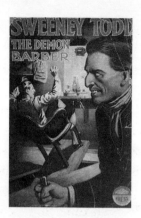

Usually the customer would land on his head and die immediately. But if he didn't, Sweeney Todd was there in a flash
with his razor. And never did a razor merit the word 'cut-
throat' more than Sweeney Todd's.

This went on for quite a while, until Sweeney Todd ran up
against a problem: what to do with the bodies.

His shop was built over some ancient catacombs – tunnels,
really – that ran under the streets, and to start with he put
the bodies there. But soon they were getting crowded: the
corpses were mounting up.

He turned to his girlfriend, Margery Lovett, for advice.
By lucky coincidence, she owned the pie shop directly across
the road from Sweeney Todd's establishment, and by a further
coincidence the two were connected via the underground
catacombs.

Margery Lovett had an idea: 'I know, Sweeney. Why don't
you butcher your customers after you've murdered them?
Then deliver the meat and innards to me via the tunnels. I can

grind it all up and put it in my pies. It'll save a fortune on my meat bill.'

Sweeney Todd scratched his head. 'Don't you think people will notice, my love?'

'Of course not, silly. I'll make lots of tasty gravy to go with them. Delicious.'

And that was what they did. They served up Sweeney Todd's customers to Margery Lovett's. And those pies were a great success with Londoners. There was a tremendous rush for the fresh ones, which came out of the oven at twelve o'clock. Here's a contemporary account: 'Oh, those delicious pies. There was about them a flavour never surpassed and rarely equalled. The paste was of the most delicate construction, and impregnated with the aroma of delicious gravy that defied description.'

Of course, Margery Lovett couldn't serve up the bones. People would have grown suspicious. So Sweeney stored them in an underground crypt.

The problem was that the flesh on those bones rotted. Above the crypt, in the church of St Dunstan's, the worshippers noticed the smell. They held perfumed handkerchiefs to their noses, but it didn't help. Eventually the rector complained, and the beadle of St Dunstan's called in the Bow Street Runners to investigate.

The Bow Street Runners were one of the world's first modern police forces, but they were always a small force. There were never more than fifteen for all of London.

When the man in charge of the Bow Street Runners, Sir

Richard Blunt, went to St Dunstan's to investigate, he smelt a rat, among other things, and his investigations soon led him in the direction of the strange barber on Fleet Street. He had some of his men stake out the shop. They soon noticed that some customers who went in for a shave didn't come out.

Then Sir Richard investigated the catacombs.

What he found there was frankly unbelievable. In one of the crypts, a pile of human remains was heaped half-way to the ceiling. Then he followed bloody footprints to Margery Lovett's basement and guessed what had been going on.

The game was up.

Margery Lovett was arrested as she was serving some of her pies. Word spread among her clientele, and she came within a hair's breadth of being lynched on the spot. When they had her safely in prison, she confessed everything, dropping Sweeney Todd in it up to his neck. Then she poisoned herself.

Sweeney Todd was arrested quietly, but his trial was sensational. The Bow Street Runners raided his home and found the clothes and sundry belongings of more than 160 men. He was one of the most prolific murderers of all time.

He never had a hope of escaping justice and was hanged in the prison yard at Newgate. By all accounts, he died hard.

So why did he do it?

Undoubtedly, robbery was a major motivator. We know that he robbed many of his victims and used the proceeds to buy himself a fine life. Also, he had been so brutalized by the time he reached adulthood that human life meant little to him. Other people were an obstacle to be removed so that he could achieve his ends.

But the pies point to something else. Someone who butchers his clients and has them made into pies must be suffering from some form of dementia. In a modern court of law, an insanity plea would probably be almost automatic.

So much for the Demon Barber. In the years after his death, he became a kind of bogeyman in England, like Jack the Ripper or Burke and Hare: a dark stain on the history of barbering. And they wrote some good songs about him.

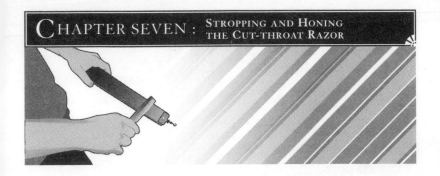

CHAPTER SEVEN : STROPPING AND HONING THE CUT-THROAT RAZOR

This chapter is all about keeping your cut-throat razor in good order. Two skills are involved: stropping and honing. Don't worry, I have diagrams that you can follow for both. They're not that hard.

STROPPING

A strop is a piece of leather that you use to keep the blade of your razor dry and correctly aligned. Even after you have wiped it with tissue paper, invisible droplets of moisture will cling to it. Stropping dries it completely.

You can't do without a strop and, anyway, it's probably the most enjoyable aspect of shaving with a cut-throat razor. You may have seen one being used in an old black-and-white movie. If you haven't, you can rent *The Great Dictator* on video and watch Charlie Chaplin doing it. But you should realize that his technique was a little flawed in parts.

Strops come in different types, shapes and sizes. When you buy a cut-throat razor, the shop will also sell you a strop as part of the deal. If they didn't it would be like selling you shoes without laces. To start off with, you can use the strop that came with your razor and it'll be fine. Later, you might want to splash out and buy the one of your choice.

THE HANGING STROP

The basic, traditional type with which most people are familiar. It's a simple strip of leather, with a piece of string or a hook at one end to hang it up.

Actually, that's not all: on many of the traditional strops, a strip of linen is attached to the top, so you have two strips fastened together. Here's a fairly typical example:

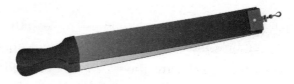

You clip a hanging strop to a hook on the wall, or a bedpost, or any other handy object. The height doesn't matter – whatever suits you. Then you hold the end and pull the razor up the smooth side – the rough side is not used – as in the diagram on p. 139.

The crucial thing to understand is that you 'pull' the blade on a strop. That means the spine of the razor leads.

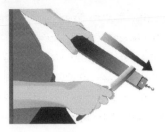

The edge trails behind. Then, when you've reached the top of the strop, you turn the blade over and pull it back down again. Again, the cutting edge trails, as below:

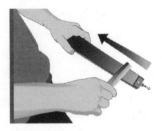

Incidentally, the grip as shown in the above diagrams is not necessarily the correct one for you. Hold your strop in whichever way feels comfortable. Make sure it's taut enough to keep the leather straight, but don't pull the hook out of the wall. Also, only use very gentle pressure on the blade. If you use too much, you risk misaligning it.

I'd better talk about the linen strop too. I'm a little wary on this point, since there's a lot of disagreement among even cut-throat-razor aficionados as to what function it serves. My theory, again based on my experience, is this: you use the linen strop first, then the leather one. You strop on both in exactly the same way. The function of the linen is to clean the blade, and also to warm it slightly, through friction, so that it's more receptive to the aligning action of the leather strop. If your strop doesn't have a linen strip attached to it, count yourself lucky that you don't have to worry about it. You can easily do without one.

THE PADDLE STROP

This is a piece of leather – or rather two pieces of leather, one on each side – glued to a wooden paddle. Here's an example:

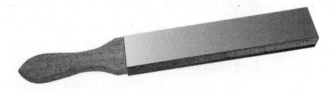

You hold it in one hand and draw the razor along its length with the other, as you would with a hanging strop. Everything is identical, including the fact that you should-n't exert too much pressure on the blade.

THE TENSION-ADJUSTABLE STROP

This strop is similar to the paddle strop, but the leather is stretched on to an iron frame. You can increase the tension by twisting the handle, which has a screw. It should

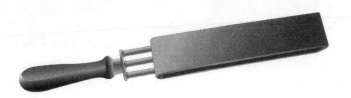

be kept fairly taut, but not so that you stretch the leather prematurely. This type of strop is normally a bit more expensive than the others.

So, which one should you choose?

It depends on your personal preference. I started off using the cheap hanging strop that came with my first razor. After a couple of years, I saw a nice tension-adjustable strop in a cigar shop in Paris. I used it for years, but now I've switched to a heavier, antique horsehide hanging strop I bought and reconditioned. I prefer a hanging strop, but they're not inherently superior to the other types. You should use whichever you have, and if you have more than one, use the one you prefer. The only advantage of a paddle or tension-adjustable strop is that you can put them into a smaller bag when travelling. You should never fold or roll a hanging strop, and if you're buying a second-hand one, avoid any whose leather has a noticeable bend: it has been stored folded. It's nearly impossible to put this right.

Razor experts might tell you differently, but all types of strop are fine. They'll keep the edge on your cut-throat correctly aligned and dry, which is all you want to achieve.

TECHNIQUE

The manner in which you strop is, however, crucial. No action defines the cut-throat-razor man more than his stropping technique, and a few things are worth mentioning here. These points hold true for all three types of strop:

- When you're turning the blade over, you turn it 180 degrees over the *spine* of the blade, not over the edge. If you turn it over the edge, you risk blunting it on the leather.

- If you strop with the edge leading, rather than trailing, you will blunt it. Also, you stand a fair chance of slicing your strop in two.

- The blade should rest lightly on the leather. Never use force. Although it may feel good, you'll misalign the blade over a period of years.

- Start off slow and increase your speed as you become more proficient. This is an activity that you're doing on your own. You're not trying to impress anyone, and if you move too fast too soon, you run the risk of a serious accident – or, worse, damaging your razor.

- How many strokes you take is a matter of personal preference. I strop about fifty times (that's twenty-five up, twenty-five down). But you probably don't need to do that many. Some people make about ten strokes each way. Some cut-throat-razor men don't have a clue how many strokes they take. They simply stop when they feel they've stropped enough, and that's a great approach to take.

- Many different types of leather are used in strops: horsehide, *rindleder* (German for 'cowhide'), sealskin and deerskin, among others. Again, different buffs will give you a list of the advantages of each type, but you shouldn't worry about that. Cow- or horsehide are probably the two that I'd go with from an ecological perspective.

People sometimes ask me what I think of when I'm shaving. The honest answer is nothing. I don't run through my daily schedule, or what I'm going to have for breakfast, or my plans for world domination. In fact, it's the opposite. I empty my mind. This is true for my shaving in general, but even more so when I strop the blade. It's one of the only times in the day when there is a complete absence of thought in my head.

MEXICAN DAYS

Let me take you back to Mexico – a place that always smelt to me of revolution: Pancho Villa, Emiliano Zapata, Leonid Trotsky – the most romantic country in the world. When I arrived, it wasn't long before I was friendly with a bunch of long-haired, unwashed, moustachioed misfits that I met on one of my first drunken nights in a shady bar. I had the same ideas as they did, and I was a long-haired misfit too.

But never unshaven.

I remember when we were all staying in an old flea-pit of a hotel in the mountains, and I was in the communal bathroom, preparing for my shave, when Carlos, one of the gang, ambled in. He turned on the tap, held his head under it, then leaned against a sink along the opposite wall, the water running on to his shirt. He pulled out a black cheroot, struck a match on his boot and held the flame to the tip. 'You gonna shave again, Blondie?'

I ran my thumb along the edge of the razor and frowned. 'Yeah.'

'This shaving thing – seems like it's a big deal for you.' He sat on the sink. His moustache drooped down the sides of his mouth.

I looked in the mirror. I could see him behind me, and heard the rasp of his hand as it passed across the three-day-old stubble on his cheeks. I pulled at a loose tile on the wall until it came away in my hands and dropped it into the neighbouring sink. It was that kind of bathroom.

'Yeah.'

I hung up my strop, turned it over to the linen side and took the tension between my fingers. I pulled the blade down the linen, flipped it over and pulled it slowly back up again. I repeated this five or six times.

I switched to the leather: heavy horsehide, gleaming from the polishing of years. I pulled the blade softly along the length and let the hiss reverberate off the walls of the bathroom.

'Most people make the mistake of applying too much

pressure when they strop. For the perfect edge, the pressure has to be light enough for that snake-hiss.'

I saw Carlos's eyes drawn to the blade as the steel hissed up its length.

'You shouldn't move too fast on the leather,' I continued. 'Do it slow and right. Let the sound of the strop relax you. Your hand needs to be relaxed for when the blade passes along your face.'

'So the sound relaxes you?'

I thought about that. 'More than relaxes. Everything becomes clearer and less complicated.'

Smoke wafted up past his face and the acrid smell hit my nose. 'And what do you think about when you're doing this, Blondie?'

'Nothing, Carlos – the opposite of thinking. It's when I flush out all the bad stuff. It's where I find peace.' I wiped the blade clean with a piece of paper.

As we stared at each other in the mirrors, he grinned. 'You want a cigar, Blondie?'

'Sure. You think I'm going to shave without one?'

STROP PASTE

Stropping is an autopilot activity. With honing, on the other hand, you have to think. Most people find honing difficult. In the beginning, I did too. I should state, though, before I start on this technique, that there is a way to avoid it. I used my cut-throat razor for years and never honed. So can you. You can use strop paste instead.

I'll explain: when you're stropping, you're not sharpening the blade. You're aligning the fin of the blade correctly, and drying it completely. However, if you use strop paste, you most definitely are sharpening the blade.

Strop paste contains very fine abrasives, which sharpen your razor as you strop. There are different varieties, and different grits. Some come in a tube, which you smear on to the strop. Some come in a block, which you rub on. To start with you use a lot to cover your strop more or less completely, but you replenish it sparingly as it wears down. You'll feel it when it's time to replenish: the blade should hiss along the surface of the strop, and it shouldn't be covered with goo when you finish.

Of course, if you're using strop paste, you'll need two strops: one covered with paste, and one plain leather. You cannot put paste on the rough side of the hanging strop – the leather is too rough. This is where a paddle strop or a tension-adjustable strop is handy. You can put paste on one side and keep the other plain. That was exactly what I did for many years. My tension-adjustable strop had a coating of cadmium oxide strop paste (the green one) on one side, and it came with a little block to replenish it when it started to wear off. This served me well, and I would never have had to change.

Eventually, though, I did change, to a fine old hanging strop. Then I bought myself a hone and went through a lot of effort and pain learning the correct technique.

Why?

For the hell of it.

Rest assured, I've used several different types of hone. They do a great job, but they're no better than strop paste. If you want the easy way out, stick with strop paste and a tension-adjustable or paddle strop. It's the idiot-proof option.

HONING

Over time, the edge of your razor will become blunted: the two edges won't meet in perfect planes any more. Your stubble wears it down, and the edge becomes rounded or jagged. Additionally, there may be dings, dents and nicks in the edge. The chances are that you won't be able to see them, unless your eyes are those of a hawk. A magnifying-glass or, even better, a microscope will help here.

To correct these imperfections, you must remove a fine layer of metal from both sides of the razor blade so that the planes meet in a perfect line again. That's what the definition of a sharp blade is: two perfect planes meeting in a perfect line.

To remove the fine layers of metal from the razor, you need a hone. You have several choices: Japanese Waterstone, Belgian Blackstone, Norton, antique barber's, ceramic, diamond abrasive . . . The list goes on and on.

If you're starting out on hones, I recommend a Norton combination 4000/8000 grit one. Grit measures the fineness of the abrasive elements. So you start off honing on the rougher 4000 grit side and finish on the finer 8000. Be warned: these are very fine grits indeed. Keep this hone for your cut-throat razor. Don't use it on kitchen knives.

You should know that most hones nowadays are man-made, not quarried. That's not a bad thing. It guarantees evenness of grit throughout the hone. You would need to be able to trust a quarried stone to use it with your cut-throat razor. If you meet a seam of something else running through it, it will play hell with your blade. Belgian Blackstone was a very famous quarried stone, but supplies are scarce.

WET OR DRY HONING

Most manufacturers recommend you use their hones with water, rather than oil, although there are some with which you can use either. If you're using water, pour it on liberally. In fact, immerse the hone for about half an hour before you start, and pour on more at intervals while you're honing. Some experts recommend that you dry-hone. That means no water or oil. They maintain that water or oil may create a paste on the hone that blunts your blade.

I've tried both wet and dry honing. I prefer dry honing. I find it gives me a better edge, and it's a lot less messy. If you're learning to hone, I recommend you try both. See which one gives you better results and run with that option.

HONING TECHNIQUE

The act of honing remains the same whether you use water or not. You push the razor with the edge first – the opposite of stropping – until you arrive at the end of the hone, then flip it *over its spine* and push it back again. It's crucial that you complete the same number of strokes on either side, and it's also crucial that you take in the whole edge of the razor in one stroke, by moving the blade in a diagonal, or curved, line across the hone. The diagram below should make it clear:

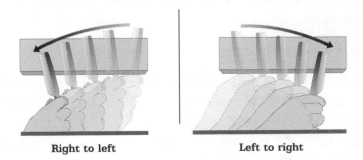

Right to left   **Left to right**

There is a way round this diagonal, curved motion. The above-mentioned Norton 4000/8000 grit hone is broad enough to fit the entire blade on it, so you can move the blade in a straight line up and down its length. That simplifies things considerably.

Probably the most important point in honing is that you keep the blade dead flat on the hone. That means the edge of the blade and the spine should touch the hone at all times. Never allow the spine to lift off the hone while the blade is travelling. If you don't adhere to this point, you'll blunt your razor and make it unusable.

Regrettably, this happened to me. The first time I honed my trusty old razor (which was perfectly sharp already from the strop paste) I blunted it. I panicked when I tried to shave with it and screamed for help from an Internet razor forum. I was given the help I needed. My problem was exactly the above: that I hadn't had the spine of the razor resting on the hone while the blade was travelling. It was a hard lesson.

The other important point is that you need only make four or five strokes each way to hone the blade. If you continue honing after this, you run the risk of developing a wire edge on the blade – a residue of metal on the very tip. You can test for this by running your fingernail over it. It will feel jagged and catchy. The way to remove a wire edge is by backhoning: dragging, rather than pushing, the edge along the hone for two or three strokes. Then you'll have to hone it all over again, taking care not to overhone this time.

That brings me to the question of how frequently to hone your razor. Some experts recommend once a month. Some say a couple of times a year. I think you should hone when you feel your razor isn't doing such a good job on your cheeks. Everyone's hair and shaving technique is different. I hone when I feel the razor beginning to drag on my stubble. This is normally about every second month.

But I also recommend honing your cut-throat razor when you're sprawled on the sofa, trying to get rid of unwelcome guests, door-to-door salesmen or politicians. To complete the effect, drool from the side of your mouth as you work.

Honing can be an acquired taste. If it doesn't suit you, or if you find it tedious, go with the strop-paste option. It's a lot easier. On the other hand, it's a nice feeling to be able to hone a razor well. And honing is a useful skill for men.

Please note, though: the honing technique described above applies to the hollow-ground cut-throat razor only. If you're honing a knife, the technique is somewhat different.

If you're interested in learning how to put an edge on all kinds of blades, there are books on it. The one I recommend is *The Razor Edge Book of Sharpening*, by John Juranitch. It doesn't deal with cut-throat razors specifically, but it gives you a very good background knowledge of the facts. It debunks a lot of old wives' tales, and makes clear that any blade can be given an edge equal to that of a razor – like an axe, for example.

HANK'S AXE

In the Canadian Rockies, a long time before Jacob Schick had thought of his electric razor, lumberjacking was a common activity. That's what Bud and Hank were doing. And they'd been doing it all summer. Now they were packing up and heading off before the cold weather hit and they were snowed in.

They were looking forward to going to town. They were eager for the relaxed company they would meet there and a few drinks in a bar. And, most of all, they were eager to see some women – the mountains could be awful lonely.

'Say, Hank.'

'Yeah?'

'You wouldn't happen to have such a thing as a razor, would you?'

Hank scratched his beard. 'Now that you mention it, I don't.'

'Damn.'

'Yeah.'

''Cause I know from experience that a woman does like a man to have his cheeks smooth sometimes.'

'Yeah.'

'Damn.'

They glanced at each other and realized they looked like a couple of wool-heads, with their beards hanging down to their shirts.

Then Bud said, 'Say, Hank.'

'Yeah?'

'You know the way you keep telling me how your axe is as sharp as any old razor?'

Hank scratched his beard some more. 'Are you seriously

thinking about using an axe to shave your face, Bud?'

'What I'm thinking, Hank, is how a woman likes to feel a man's cheek without it having a goddamned beard all over it. That's what I'm thinking.'

So Hank nodded and thought about that for a while too. Then he went to fetch his axe. He honed it a little on a stone he had, just to make sure, and then he drew his finger along the edge ever so gently. It bled, and he nodded. 'You know, this could work, Bud. Here, sit down. I'll do you first.'

About an hour later, Bud and Hank headed down the trail towards civilization, with smooth-shaven cheeks and expectations of a woman's soft hands on them.

A razor is simply a very sharp blade. If you can sharpen steel to the right degree, you can use lots of different types of blade as a razor. In 1982, in Ely, Minnesota, the above-mentioned John Juranitch set the world record for axe-sharpening and shaving: 13.5 minutes to sharpen the axe, 14 minutes to shave with it.

SUMMARY CHECKLIST

✧ Strop your blade after you shave and before if you want to.

✧ Strop slow and never use pressure.

✧ Stropping alone will not sharpen the blade. For that you need either a hone or strop paste.

✧ If you're honing, hone slow and gentle.

✧ Think twice, friend, before you use that axe on your face.

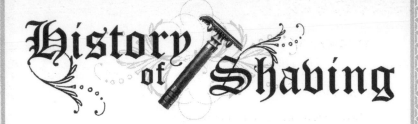

History of Shaving

THIS MODERN AGE

Here's the truth. Beards aren't acceptable now, even for peasants toiling in the fields, or their modern counterparts, workers toiling in the factories, or their ultra-modern counterparts, IT technicians toiling in call-centres.

It's understandable that women don't like beards – for physical reasons, like beard rash. But men don't like them either. Granted, you can wear one if you're a certain type of person – an Oxford professor, for example. People always make allowances for university professors. Priests and holy men get away with them too. If you're head of the United Nations you can have one (and smoke a pipe), but if you're president of the USA you can't. Benjamin Harrison was the last US president to wear a beard, in 1903, and who's ever heard of him? For businessmen, lawyers, politicians, newsreaders and the like, beards are taboo.

The reason for this shift was the First World War. Then, from a shaving perspective, two important things happened in America. First, the army needed men – to feed the enemy machine-guns mostly. The majority came from rural areas and many had beards. A lot of those beards contained lice.

The army shaved them off, willy-nilly. They cut off most of the men's hair too: the crew-cut came into its own. They justified this by saying that the gas-masks would fit better, but really it was because of the lice. America was developing its on-going obsession with hygiene, although it wasn't – and still isn't – as screwed-up in this department as the ancient Egyptians.

When the war ended, the returning soldiers were heroes, and the short-haired, clean-shaven look was in. In a few short years America had gone from a nation of beardies to a hairless one.

The other thing that happened in this period was that Gillette arrived. It was the proverbial writing on the wall for the cut-throat razor. Mr King Camp Gillette (yes, he was really called that) had recently patented his safety razor. He did a smart deal with the armed forces, and every American soldier sent off to Europe was issued with a Gillette safety razor in his backpack. When they came back, they continued to use them, of course, and Gillette made a fortune. The way men shaved had changed for ever. Now, the only men who use cut-throat razors are people like me: anarchists, oddballs and misfits.

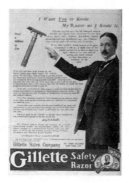

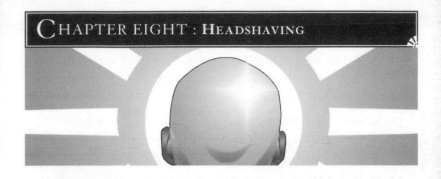

CHAPTER EIGHT : HEADSHAVING

THE MONK

In northern Thailand, Thaksin felt relaxed. He was surrounded by his entire family: mother and father, two grandparents, several brothers and sisters, aunts and uncles. He had risen early that morning and paid his respects to his ancestors. Then his family had assembled and he had knelt in front of them to bathe his elders' feet.

Now he was prepared. He seated himself on a stool and, one by one, his relatives filed past and snipped off a lock of his hair with scissors. At the same time they gave him a blessing for a prosperous future. None of the hair was allowed to fall to the ground: it was caught in a lotus leaf.

When they had finished, a monk approached. Thaksin heard the old man's chanting as if through a veil. The physical world was drifting away. The smell of incense and the chanting gave him a glimpse of his future life.

The monk started rubbing on the lather. The sun had warmed it, and it felt pleasant as it covered Thaksin's head. It smelt of oils and jasmine, and Thaksin closed his eyes, inhaling the fragrance, letting it sink into his soul.

When the lathering was done, the old monk lifted the blade, which gleamed. It was a cut-throat razor that had seen many years of service. It had shaved hundreds of heads over the course of its life, and started many souls along the path of enlightenment.

Thaksin felt the blade pass over his scalp. Where it passed, his head felt naked and cold, then light and airy, and Thaksin directed his mind towards the everlasting nature of the world, free from any physical encumbrance, towards matters that were at the centre of the universe.

Having shaved Thaksin's head, the old monk also removed his eyebrows, because they were followers of Theravada Buddhism.

Then Thaksin looked quite different. His family grouped around him again and took it in turns to pour water over him. Then they mixed herbs with the water, which turned yellow, and rubbed it into Thaksin's head and body.

After that, Thaksin had a shower and changed into his white robes. These, he would wear for one day only before changing into saffron-coloured ones.

He was nearly twenty. He would spend three months as a monk in the temple. He felt he had made a good start. His hair had been shaved off, and he would now shave away all the lower preoccupations from his heart.

THE SKINHEAD

In Sweden, Karl was sixteen. Sitting on a stool in the middle of his friends, he felt afraid. His hair fell to his shoulders. He liked it long, although his parents thought it was out of control. In fact, they thought Karl was out of control.

What do they know? Karl thought. They don't know anything about anything. He wasn't a child any more, and he was going to show them. He despised his parents for their middle-class attitudes and their weakness.

'Ready, Karl?'

Karl nodded, and his friend, Ragnar, switched on the electric clipper. With his first stroke, he carved a line right across the centre of Karl's scalp. Karl gazed into the mirror, shocked. His friends laughed. Ragnar lit a cigarette, grinned, and went to work in earnest. Karl's hair fell like sleet, and a few minutes later, his head was covered with stubble.

'You look good, Karl.'

'Yeah.'

'No more fucking hippie for you, boy.'

'No.'

'Ready for the full scalp?'

Karl didn't feel ready: he felt naked and out of his

depth. But his new friends were watching. And he knew he couldn't let them see his fear.

'I'm ready,' he said.

Ragnar picked up an aerosol can and squirted shaving cream over Karl's head. The others laughed harder. One or two joined in, rubbing it into the stubble with their fingers. Karl got some on his face and jacket.

'Right, here we go.' Ragnar picked up a disposable safety razor and went to work. It took longer than the clippers, and while Karl's head was shaved, all the others were quiet. Ragnar wasn't experienced with the blade, so there were a few uneven patches, two nicks and some razorburn. But when he had finished, Karl looked like the others.

'Now you're one of us, Karl.'

'Yeah.'

Ragnar nodded quietly. He took his cigarette out of his mouth and gave it to Karl. 'Yeah. Ready to take your place beside us in the line, Karl. Ready to stop the fucking mongrelization of the white race.'

Karl had never felt more unready in his life. His head was cold and he wanted his hair back.

THE BALDING MAN

In Chicago, despair flooded Frank Carswell. He had finished his daily shave. He splashed some water on his face, then wetted his hair and combed it.

He combed it back, as he normally did, to hide the bald patch that was spreading insidiously on top. Then he studied himself critically in the mirror. The thinning patch was safely under wraps. But his hairline seemed to be thinning too. He had noticed it a few times recently. His brow furrowed, and he took a swipe with the comb, pushing some hair sideways.

'Damn.'

That had exposed some of the top bald patch.

He took a more careful approach, dividing the strands to sweep back and to the side. He stepped away. Now he resembled some ageing punk rocker trying to shock people with his hairstyle.

'Oh, come on!'

He swept it back, but the balding patches at his temples shone. 'It's the light in this bathroom. It's too harsh.'

He walked out to the landing and looked at himself in the mirror there. Just at that moment a ray of sunlight pierced the window, and hit him straight on the head. His bald patches twinkled at him.

'Jesus, that's even worse.'

He slunk back into the bathroom, and his shoulders slumped. He had to do something. He was a successful litigation expert, with three cars and four children – all in private education. Was this the price he had to pay? He wasn't old enough to go bald. His father had died in his sixties with a full head of hair. What was going on?

He had to do something. He couldn't go on like this.

Maybe he could have implants. Maybe there was some treatment.

Then he took another look. 'Grab a hold of yourself, Mr Carswell.' He reached for the scissors.

Half an hour later, in a three-piece suit, feeling better than he had felt in a long time, he went down to breakfast. Mary was already back from driving the children to school and was clearing away the breakfast things.

'Oh, my God! Frank?'

Frank smiled and opened his arms. 'Well, what's the verdict?'

Mary stared at her husband's gleaming, clean-shaven head. Was this really him? He looked younger, leaner, sexier.

Mary hesitated, then smiled back. 'Yeah, you look good. I like it.'

MOTIVATIONAL FACTORS

People shave their heads for a variety of reasons. The above stories are only a few examples. Ask a prisoner in some of the tougher countries of the world. He had it done when he was arrested. He had no choice in the matter.

Swedish Karl did his out of a need to belong. The skinhead movement was always kind of strange and shaving the head is a rite of passage into the group. Long hair is associated with the sixties free-love and marijuana against which they reacted violently. By the way, it should be noted that not all European skinheads are Fascists.

Thaksin, our friend from Thailand, had only limited choice in the matter. Thai men are not considered mature until they've spent time as a Buddhist monk. In fact, if you work for the Thai government, you're allowed to take three months' paid leave to be a monk. Many private companies in Thailand allow this too. Until you've done your stint, you're considered an 'unripe' man.

As for Frank, the American lawyer, there are legions of middle-aged Franks who have experienced at least one panic attack at the signs of impending baldness. For many of these men, disguising the bald patch with a comb-over is a knee-jerk reaction.

In the end, Frank took the honourable way out. He didn't have to shave it all off, of course. He could have merely clipped it short. In this regard, there are a few points you should know about male-pattern baldness:

- Baldness is hereditary, and passes through your mother's line. If you're a young man and want to know if you're going to go bald or not, look at your mother's side of the family. It's her X-chromosome that determines your future hairline.
- Baldness is a sign of masculinity. Men instinctively react to bald men on a different level.
- Baldness is a sign of virility. It means your sex drive is still going strong.

- Never comb your hair over a bald patch — it will expose you to an incredible amount of ridicule among your fellow men.
- Never wear a wig. That will expose you to even more ridicule. Which is completely deserved.

HOW TO SHAVE YOUR HEAD

Whatever the reason, let's assume you've decided to do it.

How do you start?

First, I recommend you to go to a barber and have a crew-cut: half an inch or less. Alternatively, buy yourself an electric hair clipper and do it yourself. Starting at about half an inch or less is definitely the clever move here.

A friend of mine went to a barber once and asked him to shave it all off. The barber refused point-blank. He gave him a half-inch cut and a tube of oil, with the following advice: 'Your scalp is flaky and dry, sonny. If I shave it clean, you'll look like a leper. They won't let you into the pub. Rub that oil in for a week, then come back and I'll finish the job.'

That kind of advice can be invaluable before you take the big step. And let's be absolutely clear on this: you're taking a big step. Hair grows on average less than half an inch per month. It will take a long time to grow back.

You also need to be prepared for people's reactions to

a shaved head. If you're in Thailand, wearing a saffron robe, it's not a problem: people understand where you're coming from. But in Western Europe or North America people might form the idea that you're one of Karl's blood-brothers.

But let's assume you have your half-inch cut. Now rub your hand over your scalp a couple of times. Can you feel any bumps, dents or irregularities? If you can, be prepared for them to become highly visible when you shave it all off. The number-one reason that a balding man doesn't shave it all off is because his head is an irregular shape, or because it has irregularities – i.e. bumps.

If you're still decided on taking it off, though, start lathering. There's no mystery about shaving your head. You proceed in the same way as you do when you shave your face. Showering, lathering, softening, shaving brushes and high-quality shaving cream all hold as true for your head as they do for your face. You can use an electric razor, if you prefer.

In fairness, I should mention that a couple of razors are designed specifically for headshaving. The main difference between them and a normal safety razor is the shape, which is intended to make it easier to hold as you shave. I haven't tried these, but you can look them up on the Internet. Do a websearch for:

- Headblade
- Dovo Headshaver

Shave your head in stages: lather and shave the front first, then the sides and the back. As with any job, breaking it down into segments will make it easier.

Once you've done the deed and it's all off, you'll probably notice a few things.

My head looks deathly white in comparison to my face (if you're Caucasian).

This is normal: hair has protected your scalp from nearly all sunlight for most of your life. Whatever you do, don't go out in the sun and try to get a tan. Your scalp can burn very badly. The difference in tone will probably disappear over a couple of weeks, provided you keep shaving your head.

My head is a funny shape. And what about all those bumps?

I tried to warn you about this one. Some men's heads look good when they're bald. Others' don't. Tough luck if you're not happy with the result. Grow back whatever hair you can.

My head feels cold.

This isn't really true. Yes, it feels cool, but that will wear off in a few days, or even a few hours. However, you should invest in a hat, or even a couple. Apart from anything else, even a shower of rain will be irritating if it's pattering on your bald head. A hat will also protect you against direct sunlight. And hats fit bald men better than they do hairy men.

My head is really shiny. How can I reduce that?

There are special moisturizing creams designed to reduce shininess on your face and you can use them on your head too. Alternatively, don't shave so close next time, or don't shave so frequently. A bit of stubble will take the shine right off. Do not attempt to reduce the shine by rubbing with sandpaper, a Brillo pad or any other abrasive.

My head isn't as shiny as I want it to be. How can I increase that?

Shave very close next time. Also, ironic as it sounds, slap some hair pomade on it. Rub it in well. Massaging your bald scalp with pomade feels great.

THE TURKISH BARBER OF MALTA

I've had a half-inch and less many times, but a full shave only once.

I was training in Malta. It was midsummer, and I had just finished a long run and was covered with sweat. While I was making my way back to the hotel, through a winding street in the old city of Valletta, I stopped and stared: I was outside a gem of a barbershop: red leather seats, gold-framed mirrors, bric-à-brac hanging off the ceiling, Turkish music drifting out of the open door. An enormous bald man with a handlebar moustache beamed out at me. How could I resist?

I slung my bag into a corner and eased myself into the window-seat.

He looked at me and said something in Turkish or Maltese – I couldn't tell the difference. I wiped my hand across my brow and held up the sweat for him to see, then pointed at my hair. 'It's too hot. Make it shorter.'

The moustache grinned. 'Good.'

Then I spotted the cut-throat razors on the shelf, the horsehide strop, the shaving brushes. I knew that I was in the company of a traditional Turkish barber. I rubbed my hand over my chin and pointed at the razors. 'And a shave.'

Again, the moustache grinned at me. 'Good, good.'

He tilted the chair back a fraction, then spun it playfully while he started his preparations, singing something that sounded like the Turkish Song of the Damned. I was left staring at the whirling ceiling, laughing.

He stopped the chair before I was too dizzy. He had washed his hands and was standing by my side with the shaving bowl. He started to lather my neck, worked up along my cheeks, finishing off around my chin and nose. I caught the distinctive scent of crushed almond.

Then he went back to the sink and turned on a steaming tap, drenched several towels and wrung them out. As he folded them over my face, I could feel the tension slipping away. He had the temperature exactly right.

When he had finished with the last fold over my eyes, I was completely relaxed. I heard the gentle, rhythmic hissing as he drew his razor along the strop.

Now, at that point I did something you should never do. It may have been the heat, the soothing Turkish music, the scent of crushed almonds . . . Who knows? The fact is, I fell asleep.

When I woke, it was to feel my face being patted down with talc. I blinked and stared at the ceiling. The handle-bar moustache loomed over me. 'Good?'

Something felt very wrong. My head was cold. I sat up and faced the mirror.

I was spear-bald.

'Christ almighty!'

'Good?'

I ran my fingers over the naked expanse of my skull. It gleamed white and smooth as glass. How had he done it without waking me up?

He sensed something was amiss, and his smile dropped a fraction. 'Not good?'

He must have had the deftest touch I had ever encountered. The fact that I hadn't wanted to be bald was irrelevant. The man had shaved my entire head without waking me, and that's skill of the highest order.

'Uh . . . very good. Thank you.'

I paid him his money, picked up my bag and shuffled off down the street to look for a hat.

Then I grew my hair back, inch by inch.

Summary Checklist

+ If you're wondering whether you'll go bald, don't look at your father. Instead, check the hairline of your mother's brothers.

+ Don't try to disguise your impending baldness. Wear those bald patches with pride.

+ If you're going to take the big step, be advised that it takes a long time to grow back. Go for a crew-cut first and see how you like it.

+ Saffron robes don't look good on Westerners.

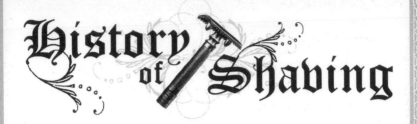

History of Shaving

BEARDED REVOLUTIONARIES

After the First World War, America was clean-shaven. Beards were out for the army, the marine corps, the navy, the police forces, nearly all large corporations and government agencies. From the 1920s to the 1960s beards were bad in America. In fact, beards were practically Communist.

That last crack about Communists is true. Although Mao Tse-tung was a very hairless man, Karl Marx and Friedrich Engels both had massive beards. Lenin had a goatee and so did Trotsky. Stalin had a moustache so enormous it nearly counted as a beard, and even Ho Chi Minh sported a long flowing goatee. Mussolini, a truly hairless Fascist, went so far as to state: 'I am anti-whiskers. Fascism is anti-whiskers.'

True, Nikita Khrushchev was all-round bald as an egg, but the arch-villain — that Cuban devil — right on America's doorstep: he had a goddamned enormous beard.

That's right: Fidel Castro. And his comrade Che Guevara had one too, albeit a straggly affair that didn't even cover his cheeks, but that wasn't for lack of trying.

I must admit that Fidel and Che are some of my all-time heroes. There were even times in my life when I grew a beard in sympathy with the revolution.

CUBA

Fidel met up with Che in Mexico. His first insurgency had already failed, and Che tagged along for the ride when Fidel went back to Cuba for another try. They had about eighty men with them when they landed, but Batista's troops ambushed them. In no time at all, there were only seventeen left. They took off to the hills – the Sierra Maestra. Batista sent an army up against them, but they fought hard, and most of the peasants supported them, so they survived.

Then, one day, they found themselves pinned down by enemy fire. Che and Fidel were crouched behind an old log, bullets whistling through the air. Things looked grim.

Fidel pulled out a cigar – one of his last. It was an H. Upmann, in case anyone's interested; he smoked Cohibas later on, but they hadn't been invented yet, so at this time he smoked Upmanns, Bauzas, Trinidads, Partagas, whatever he could lay his revolutionary hands on. When you're holed up in the jungle with government troops trying to blow your head off, I suppose you smoke what you can get.

Che lit up a Tabaco cigar. 'Hey, Fidel, I've been meaning to ask you something.'

'Sure.'

'It looks like you've stopped shaving.'

Fidel rubbed his cheeks. 'I ran out of razor blades a while back.'

'I can lend you one if you want.'

'No.' Fidel shook his head. 'In fact, I think this might be a good look for us.'

Che scratched his head. 'You're kidding, right?'

'Listen, Che. We need to rebel against every part of society – even the goddamned shaving system. This could make us as revolutionaries.'

Che rubbed his cheeks. 'That's bullshit, Fidel. You've got a decent growth on your face, but mine's all straggly. I'll look like shit.'

'Che, if you just stop shaving, I predict that you'll become the premier face of revolutions everywhere. Millions of teenagers will have your photograph on their bedroom walls. Your face will be an icon.'

Che thought about this. 'Hey, you think the women will go for it?'

'Sure. You'll get laid all the time.'

Che, who had a really crazy streak, shrugged. 'OK, I'll give it a try. But if I don't get laid, I'm shaving it off again. Now, let's get the hell out of here.'

With cigars and guns blazing, fuelled by the courage endowed by their growing beards, they fought their way out from behind that log, toppled Batista's rotten dictatorship, took over Cuba and firmly entrenched the beard as a rebel fashion statement.

Years later, Che was murdered in Bolivia, but Fidel Castro

became the patron of the Whiskers Club in Derbyshire, England, having promised not to shave off his two-year-old beard until his country had a 'good government'. Then he nearly precipitated a nuclear war in the Cuban missile crisis.

The USA, of course, was enraged by Fidel and his revolution, and successive presidents authorized the CIA to either assassinate or discredit the man they codenamed 'the beard'.

Most of you have probably heard the poison-cigar story, but one of the more fiendish of the CIA's schemes was to dust the inside of Fidel's shoes with thallium powder. Thallium salts are a depilatory. What they were aiming for with that scheme was not to kill him, but to make his beard fall out and hence discredit him as a revolutionary leader.

MANDELA

In South Africa, Nelson Mandela, in his revolutionary days, was even more attached to his beard than Fidel. In fact, his beard was one of the reasons he was caught and slammed into jail for twenty-seven years. Here's an excerpt from an interview with one of his revolutionary buddies, who tried to keep the man alive while he was on the run from the police: 'His [Mandela's] photographs had appeared and this beard was very well known. We had suggested that he should shave off that beard. He refused. He just refused . . . the beard he would not cut. And that beard went with him to Algeria. If you see that photograph . . . in the training camp in Algeria, he's got the beard. He came back with the beard. He was arrested with Cecil Williams [with the beard].'

Nelson Mandela went through a lot in that prison. But it was only after twenty-seven years that the beard was well and truly gone and he emerged, victorious, as one of the great statesmen of our times.

THE SIXTIES

With those revolutionary examples, the beard became an anti-establishment statement. In the sixties, young men throughout the West threw away their razors, pulled on faded jeans and grew their hair to their shoulders. They smoked marijuana and listened to music their parents thought was meaningless noise. They had sex all over the place and didn't even have the decency to be ashamed of it. Western civilization was on the brink of collapse.

While they blazed a trail for sexual freedom, their musical leaders were slow to follow suit with beards, although Jimi Hendrix grew a moustache. But the Rolling Stones and the Monkees remained clean-shaven. True, John Lennon in his love-in with Yoko Ono had a bushy beard, and Jim Morrison grew one when he started doing heroin, putting on weight and generally going to pieces. But, in general, the beard made a political, not a musical statement.

The Reaction

Establishment figures found it outrageous that their stoned, degenerate sons weren't shaving. And they reacted. Beards were ruled out of bounds in most major companies – there are still some, in this day and age, that won't let you grow a beard, for no particular reason other than that they're vaguely against the revolution. And shaving – or not shaving – has become a political activity. I worked for a multinational corporation once where you were permitted to have a beard, but not to grow one. You had to acquire it during your holidays.

Police forces across America, the army and the marine corps banned beards, and still do; the navy allowed them for a period in the 1970s and 1980s, then banned them again. In the British Royal Navy, you can have a 'full set', a beard and moustache together, but not a beard or a moustache. God only knows why. In the other branches of the military, you're allowed a moustache only. The exceptions to this rule are Pioneer warrant officers, and colour sergeants. With them, beards are traditional, as also with the Beefeaters. Sikhs, of course, are allowed beards.

The battle of the beards has been well and truly lost. The beardies' last hurrah was in the eighties, when Don Johnson in *Miami Vice* persuaded hordes of us to grow designer stubble. But even that was short-lived. The present is clean-shaven. Who knows what the future will bring?

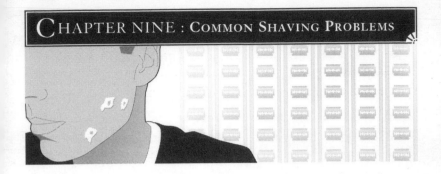

For most men, shaving should not be painful. If you follow even some of the advice in this book, it will be a positive experience. When I have time I quite enjoy shaving.

But some men have serious problems with it, and I'm about to offer some advice on how to deal with them. I want to stress two things :

- I have no direct experience in this area. Shaving for me has never been a problem. Therefore, I have gathered from other people, who are experts in these matters, the information I'm presenting in this chapter.
- If you have a serious problem with shaving, you should seek medical advice. A dermatologist (skin specialist) is the person to consult.

ACNE

Most of us have experienced acne in our teenage years.

As puberty sets in, a boy's body produces increased amounts of testosterone, with a range of effects. From a psychological perspective, he manifests bizarre behaviour: rebelliousness, driving his parents and teachers up the walls, listening to loud music and smoking behind the bike shed. He also becomes very sexually alive, which is great, and leads to more forbidden activities behind the bike shed.

From a physical perspective, he starts to grow hair in the strangest places. And the sebaceous glands produce more sebum, a fancy term for a kind of oil. So teenagers have oily skin. We all know that.

The problem is that the sebum may block the openings on your skin called follicles and cause a range of problems:

- Whiteheads are enlarged and plugged hair follicles beneath the skin. They appear as white spots.
- Blackheads are enlarged and plugged hair follicles that have reached the surface of the skin. They appear as black spots.
- Pimples occur when infection sets in. They appear as yellow spots.
- A cyst is a deep, pus-filled lesion that is painful and can cause scarring.

How much acne you have is determined largely by heredity. But other factors may play a part too, like stress, diet, tight-fitting clothes and teenage boys' notorious aversion to soap and water.

So how does acne relate to shaving?

Shaving is a recognized method of exfoliating, and it can help unblock clogged follicles. You can shave, gently, over whiteheads and blackheads, which may help reduce acne. But be careful: shaving is not a cure for acne and should not be seen as such. And there are a few points to take on board.

First, you should be using a sharp blade. A blunt one may aggravate acne. That means you should change your safety razor after three or four shaves. Also, I don't recommend you use a multi-blade safety razor if you have acne, since you'll be going over the same area many times, which can irritate and inflame your skin. I recommend that you stick with one pass, going with the grain of the beard.

Shaving over pimples is generally a bad idea. It hurts and you'll probably bleed. If you have many, proceed gently. Try, as far as possible, to skirt them when you shave. If some areas of your face are covered with pimples, don't shave them until they have cleared, at least partially.

When you have finished the shave, it's important to pat your face dry with a clean towel. Don't rub. This is a basic precaution against spreading bacteria (*propionibacterium acnes*) all over your face.

Try shaving with an electric and a safety razor, and see which feels better on your skin. Go with the one that's most comfortable. Whichever you use, make sure you keep it clean.

Avoid all alcohol-based aftershaves. Some people believe that you should use alcohol to dry out the skin, which will clear up pimples. This is a myth. Use a dermatologist-approved, oil-free moisturizer after shaving. The technical term here is *non-comedogenic*, which means that it won't clog your pores. There is also an antibiotic product called Dalacin T solution, which dermatologists frequently prescribe. You should definitely avoid using alum or talc, since they can clog the follicles.

Apart from this, the best advice I can give you on shaving with acne is the same as I have offered in the other chapters of this book: give yourself the most comfortable shave you can. Irritating the skin is to be avoided. That means, too, that you shouldn't shave every day. Most teenagers don't need to anyway (apart from the gorilla who stole my girl at the school disco).

RAZOR BUMPS

The common term for *pseudofolliculitis barbae*. This is a common condition among men with wiry, curly hair, especially black men. It's also very painful. When you shave the hair off at skin level, it may grow out, then curl directly into the skin. The diagram on p. 181 should make this clear:

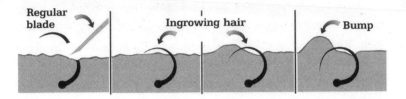

The 'bumps' appear as tender, raised spots. They can become infected and are sometimes mistaken for acne. If you're not sure whether they're acne or razor bumps, consult a dermatologist.

Razor bumps can be a problem on either the face or the head. Obviously, shaving over them is painful. There are various different products and techniques that you can try.

The basic precaution here is to avoid irritating the skin. Use a single-blade razor. Don't be concerned about achieving a very close shave: that is what causes razor bumps in the first place. Stick to one pass, and don't shave against the grain. Don't overstretch the skin while shaving, as this can lead to a very close shave, which will exacerbate the problem.

Some men advocate using an electric razor, but others say it makes the problem worse. Try an electric razor and a wet shave and see which works best for you. Go with the more comfortable alternative.

Use an exfoliating cleanser once or twice a week: it helps rid the skin of dead cells and may also free trapped hair.

You can try using a clean, soft-bristled toothbrush, or a clean, rough facecloth, in combination with a facial cleanser. Rub the toothbrush or facecloth *gently* over the affected areas. This should free up the hairs lodged in the skin.

If you have razor bumps, don't shave over them. Dislodge the hairs from the skin and wait until the inflammation has passed before you shave.

Dalacin T solution is also prescribed frequently by dermatologists for razor bumps. It has a very high success rate.

PRODUCTS

A range of specialist products is available for men who suffer from razor bumps.

Bump Fighter make a razor designed not to go too close to the skin. Several companies produce specially formulated aftershaves to treat razor bumps. Do a web-search for:

- Bump Patrol
- Bump Down
- Bump Fighter
- Bump No More

Most work by sloughing off some of the outer skin and attack the structure of the hair so that it can't curl back into the skin.

If none of the above works for you, there are two other things you can try.

Depilatories

Remember the ancient Egyptians with their arsenic depilatory cream, or the Romans with powdered viper?

Since then things have moved on. Products like Magic Shave or Nair incorporate a range of chemicals to remove unwanted hair. If shaving really isn't working for you, even with all of the above advice, you can investigate some of the modern depilatories. But I recommend talking to a dermatologist before you do so.

Lasers

Great-uncle Hector's vision of the future has come to pass. But laser hair removal is a drastic step. It's designed to be permanent. The laser beam hits the pigment in the hair follicle. The hair should then fall out and won't be able to grow back. For this one, you definitely need to talk to a dermatologist, and you should probably have tried all other options first.

Acne and razor bumps are the two most serious conditions you can face with shaving. But there are minor ones too. I've put together a chart you can flick through. If you don't find the answer there, you should seek medical help.

Problem	Probable cause	Advice
Shaving is painful. My hair feels like it's being pulled out by the roots.	You're using a blunt blade, or you haven't softened your stubble enough.	Sharpen your cutthroat or buy a new disposable razor. Shave after a hot shower and use a shaving brush with a high-quality cream.
I'm left with patches of stubble after my shave.	You're using a blunt blade, or you're rushing it. You may also be angling your blade too steeply.	Use a sharp blade. Take your time and make sure you maintain a 30-degree angle at all times.
I frequently nick myself while shaving.	You may be using a blunt blade. It's possible that you haven't softened your stubble enough, or you may be too tense while shaving. Also, you may not be tautening your skin sufficiently.	Relax. Keep a loose grip on the razor. Use a sharp blade and make sure you soften your stubble sufficiently. Make sure your skin is taut on every stroke.

PROBLEM	PROBABLE CAUSE	ADVICE
My neck is very tender. I always have razor-burn/ red spots/nicks there.	In fact, your neck probably isn't more tender than anywhere else. The problem is that you're shaving against the grain there.	Remember that your neck hair may grow in different directions. Take time to find out which way the grain goes. Shave with the grain on your first pass.
I always seem to nick/irritate myself in the same spot.	You may have a sensitive spot. Or the stubble may be tougher there, or growing in a different direction.	Make sure you're going with the grain. Also, leave that troublesome spot for last and lather it again just before you shave it.
No matter what I do, the shave irritates and inflames my skin.	Apart from all of the above advice, you may have an allergy to a product you're using. Many men have mild allergies they're not even aware of.	Try using no aftershave product for a week. If that doesn't help, try changing your pre-shave product for a week. See if the problem disappears.

PROBLEM	PROBABLE CAUSE	ADVICE
I suffer from razor-burn.	You may be shaving across or against the grain on the first pass. You may be taking short, choppy strokes in all directions.	Take longer, smoother strokes, with the grain. If you're tempted to go across or against it, wait until you've lathered again.
I just hate shaving. It really bothers me that men have to do this.	You're not one of life's natural shavers.	Grow a beard.

That last piece of advice is no joke. If you've really had it with shaving – if it's not for you – then you may be one of the minority who still have the willpower to man the barricades against the encroaching effeminization of the male.

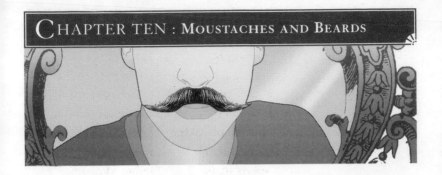

CHAPTER TEN : MOUSTACHES AND BEARDS

H ere's a joke I heard recently.

Jack, a married man, is at a three-day business conference. He's been trying to have an affair with one of his colleagues for quite a while, and she finally agrees, but only if he shaves off his beard: she thinks facial hair is horrible.

So he shaves it off, and enjoys his reward.

The following night, Jack returns home to his wife, who's already in bed, asleep. He cuddles up to her, guilty conscience and all, and rubs his now smooth chin against the back of her neck.

'Oh, Matthew,' she croons, 'you feel wonderful, but you shouldn't be here. Jack's due home tonight.'

Psychoanalysts could have a whale of a time with that joke. In some schools of psychoanalysis, shaving is seen as a form of auto-castration that men go through daily to quell their Oedipal desires.

I think that Jack had no such thing in mind. He shaved his beard off for sex. That's the reason we all shave it off.

A lot of women don't like beards, and if you grow one, you're going against their wishes.

Then again, that might be an oversimplification. In several studies, bearded men have been rated as more masculine, aggressive, mature, independent, strong and dominant. Those would all seem to be good things, right? But in the same studies, none of the bearded men was chosen as a possible mate. So, it may be that women like the look of them, but don't want to cosy up to them.

If you grow a beard, you're also going against the wishes of society. Beards are almost completely outlawed in politics. After the 2000 American presidential débâcle, Al Gore took time off for a deserved break in the sun. When he came back, he was wearing what I thought was a rather dashing beard. His picture was on the front page of most American newspapers, with all kinds of speculation as to whether he was permanently leaving politics, and further speculation as to whether he was an all-time loser.

But the tide may be turning. The Beard Liberation Front (BLF) is trying to counteract this pernicious state of affairs. It works hard to defeat the idea that 'beardies are weirdies'. They support legal action against beard discrimination and recently put on a mass beard-wagging protest in London.

But even with the BLF, many men can't face the thought of growing a full face of hair, and that leads us into the partial-beard area: a place where preconceptions, stereotypes and hidden meanings lurk.

Sideburns were originally named burnsides, after General Ambrose E. Burnside, a Union general in the American civil war with a truly impressive pair. After a while, though, people forgot about him and decided that the syntax of burnsides was all wrong and rechristened them 'sideburns'. They are also known as muttonchops, sidewhiskers or dundrearys, depending on how far they reach towards your mouth. In fact, some men go the whole distance and let them form a continuous line with the moustache.

Sideburns have a distinguished history. They were a great favourite with British colonels in the days of the Charge of the Light Brigade and the Raj. How ironic, then, that many military forces now limit the extent of the sideburn to the lower earlobe. Colonel Blimp would have had a fit.

Along with the decline of the Raj, sideburns disappeared for many years. And then, one fine day, Elvis Presley burst on to the stage with a completely new take on the colonel's whiskers. Elvis's glossy sideburns had nothing to do with tradition or the military. Like Valentino in a previous age, they were about sex. He wiggled his hips in fantastic directions and drove women berserk. And teenage boys across the land grew their sideburns long, in hope and expectation.

Elvis's sideburns developed with his persona. As he

aged, they expanded, until they covered a sizeable area of his cheeks. Even when he heeded Liberace's advice, and paraded around in gold-sequinned jumpsuits, he still drove women berserk. I put it down to the sideburns.

Now Elvis's influence has waned, and people grow sideburns to make their own personal statement, which can be tailored, depending on how you tailor your sideburns. A long, thin line running down to your jawline looks sharp, intelligent and sophisticated. A protruding, bushy growth makes a man look ape-like, primitive, uncontrolled. A trimmed, zigzag line across the lower cheek looks downright idiotic. But no matter which way you grow them, sideburns carry a whiff of sexuality and subversion.

They can be handy if you're cursed with a long, narrow face: they may make it seem broader. They can also disguise protruding ears (but they have to be really bushy for that). And if you have very bushy sideburns, your lover may grab them with both hands in a moment of passion, which, I'm reliably informed, is very painful.

THE MOUSTACHE

During my time in the Middle East, I noticed that nearly every single man had a moustache (beards, contrary to Western preconceptions, aren't common). The best curse I heard there was: 'May the fleas of a thousand camels infect your moustache, and may your arms grow too short to scratch them.'

Southern India is the same. The moustache is everywhere: it's a symbol of manhood. In fact, until quite recently there was a notorious Indian bandit, called Veerappan, who epitomized the moustache as a virility symbol in the Tamil Nadu province. His was a drooping affair of epic proportions. He eluded several successive police forces sent to terminate him and was accused of complicity in more than a hundred murders. One of his victims was a former state minister. He also kidnapped a famous Indian film star. At one point, more than two thousand police were combing the forests for him and he still managed to escape.

When his end came in a hail of bullets, people were unsure whether it was really him. His enormous moustache had been reduced to a fraction of its former glory. It emerged that just before the fatal ambush he had trimmed it to avoid recognition and capture.

In the West, the moustache has a strong history and a weak present. Once there were myriad styles. You could have it drooping over the sides of your mouth. Or you could apply moustache wax and turn up the ends for a 'Kaiser', named after Kaiser Wilhelm II of Prussia. The Kaiser moustache was generally large, and men wore a hair-net over it while they slept to keep it in shape. You could buy dinky little combs for them too.

The handlebar moustache, of which Lord Kitchener's

was the most famous example, was a monstrous growth. Originally military, it has long since crossed over into motorcycle gangs and gay bars. But it was a little imprac- tical, and in its heyday, china manufacturers designed a special cup that would keep it dry as you drank. The walrus moustache was of similar proportions to the handlebar, but with drooping ends. If you're attracted to these larger specimens, be warned: a handlebar or a walrus is a hazard if you find yourself in a bar-room brawl. If you're ever grabbed by the moustache, the expe- rience can redefine your concept of pain.

The last I should mention here is the 'toothbrush', or simply the 'Chaplin'. Chaplin's moustache defined the man. His genius in both humour and pathos is unshake- ably linked to the furry growth on his upper lip. Possibly because of its uniqueness, it did not inspire many imita- tors. Men might admire Chaplin, but they didn't want to look like him.

And then, of course, there was Hitler.

Many people assume that Hitler's moustache was a copy of Chaplin's. This is not true. Hitler wore a full han- dlebar moustache during the First World War (he fought in the trenches). He converted the handlebar to a tooth- brush probably for reasons of practicality and changing fashion.

Chaplin was both a humane and consistently left-wing man. He despised Hitler, and filmed and self-financed *The Great Dictator* – in the teeth of much opposition from

Hollywood – in order to parody him. The film was a success on all fronts. But the Battle of the Toothbrush was lost. Because of Hitler, the 'Chaplin' moustache disappeared after the Second World War. To this day it remains the only facial hair that is taboo for men.

THE GOATEE

The goatee is diabolic. There's no other name for it. The devil is routinely depicted wearing a goatee. He inherited this style from the god Pan, who enjoyed outrageous drunkenness with satyrs and nymphs and generally carrying on. Pan had a spectacular goatee, since he was half goat anyway. Old horror films routinely depict evil masterminds wearing them. The 'Fu Manchu', named after a fictional Chinese master criminal, is an exaggerated goatee/moustache combination. Clever, sophisticated, over-educated men, intellectuals, professors, jazz musicians and actors, wear goatees. And everyone knows that these types turn frequently to the dark side, with their goatees helping them along the way.

Strictly speaking, the goatee is a tuft of hair at the end of the chin, and its name derives from the billy goat, which sports a similar tuft. But men with goatees frequently grow a moustache round the mouth also. The correct term for this is a 'Vandyke'.

There are advantages to this type of beard. A goatee

may disguise a receding or double chin. It will make your face appear longer and more pointed, so roundy-cheeked men sometimes wear them. It can also make you look more intelligent, so idiots wear them too. In fact, the greatest single danger of a goatee is that it will fool people into believing that you're smarter than you are. You run the risk of being given work you're incapable of performing. I speak from experience here. I used to have a goatee.

THE FULL BEARD

There are two types of men with full beards: those who grow one to see how it looks, and those who are in it for the long haul.

The long-haulers are an exceptional bunch. I take my hat off to them. They may have a physical reason for growing a beard – like sensitive skin – but most just want a beard, and are strong enough to resist substantial pressure to remove it.

The short-termers are people like me. One day I look in the mirror and notice I haven't shaved for a few days, and the stubble is coming along nicely.

'To hell with it,' I say. 'I'm gonna be a hairy wild man now.'

These temporary beards last less than a year. Eventually the razor comes out and the beard comes off.

That's another reason I like using a cut-throat. With an electric or a safety, you would have to use scissors or an electric clipper to trim it before shaving. Not with a cut-throat: you simply lather the beard and slash through the jungle.

The temporary beard can make you look wild, Bohemian, sexual, revolutionary, shaggy, tough, mature and deep.

It can also make you look like a half-wit.

It all depends on what kind of a face and what kind of facial hair you have.

First, be warned: if you're growing a beard, it will go through an annoying, itchy stage. The timeframe on this will vary, but it can last from one to ten weeks. After that, it should have grown out. If it's your first time, rest easy: beards are not permanently itchy.

GROOMING

It's a good idea to take care of your beard. Sharp scissors and a comb should be enough for most, but you can put oil or cream on it too to take out some of the curls. You should wash it as often as the hair on your head, or it may start to stink. It may be a good idea to use conditioner on it, since facial hair is wiry.

The final grooming point is related to defining your beard. Most beards look a lot better if you shave the lower part of your neck. There's a natural line running along your neck, where the face ends and the neck begins. This is sometimes called a 'neck line' or a 'beard line'. If you shave it, it will make your beard look tidier and defined. Some men may not want the tidy look, and if you plan to grow your beard down to your chest, it will obscure your neck anyway.

A full beard will hide bad skin. It will hide fat cheeks, a double or receding chin. It will hide warts and scars. In fact, it will hide half your damn face. It will also keep your face warm (relatively) if you're unfortunate enough to be caught in a hurricane on a fishing-boat in the northern Atlantic.

On the negative side, beards are flammable. This might sound like a joke, but it's not. It's quite easy for a stray candle, match or cigar to obliterate a beard. Be vigilant.

PERSONAL EXPERIENCES

In my student years, I had a fine drooping moustache, with long hair to match. I thought it made me look like a ferocious Visigoth ready to charge the Roman lines. In fact, I probably looked awful since I'm fair-haired and moustaches don't look good on fair-haired people (but beards are OK).

Later, I went through my diabolic stage, and grew a

goatee. In fact, I had it on my wedding day, with the pictures to prove it.

Later still, I wore a full beard as I retreated deeper and deeper into ancient libraries, but that, too, went under the razor.

As I write this book, I'm wearing my all-time favourite: Soul-patch, Attilio, Royale, Imperiale, Mouche (French for fly), flavour saver, ball-tickler, womb broom, lip goatee. They all describe the same thing: a tuft of hair under the lower lip. This one was in favour with the French officer corps in their days of empire. Recently, it reappeared with Californian surfers and all kinds of new-age tribalists.

I love it. You can twirl it between your fingers. It separates you from the common herd. It's distinguished. It's so goddamn great that everyone should have one.

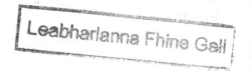

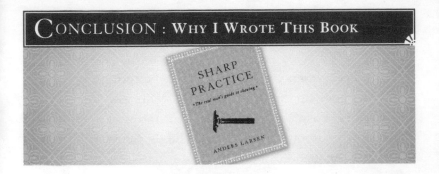

CONCLUSION : WHY I WROTE THIS BOOK

Writing this book was hard, and there were times when I asked myself why I was doing it. I came up with two answers:

- I wanted to talk about fathers and sons.
- I wanted to help.

FATHERS AND SONS

In the course of research, I've talked to different people about how men learn how to shave nowadays. The men agreed that most of us go through what I went through on my first shave: pain and bleeding, poor-quality materials and a general teenage cluelessness as regards technique. The women were a little surprised: 'Why don't your fathers teach you?'

I was stumped for an answer to that one, and in the end I put it down to the teenage-rebellion thing. At that age you're probably not getting on too well with your father.

So here's some parental advice, for what it's worth.

Fathers: when you notice your son sprouting that fuzz on his upper lip, don't be afraid to volunteer some help, even if he hasn't talked to you in three weeks (because you won't let him have a motorbike). Shaving is scary when it's your first time.

Sons: ask your father to help you out with your first shave. Even if he hasn't talked to you for three weeks (because you wrecked his car), it's worthwhile communicating on this one. Shaving, unlike everything else under the sun, is something he really does know how to do better than you.

But if neither of you is feeling up to the teacher/ student relationship, you can still try this.

When my father was sixteen, his father took him down to the local barbershop. While he was being lathered for the first time, he also gave him his first cigar. They sat there, laughed and talked together, while my father smoked and had his first shave.

I think that's a good thing to share with one another. And there are still plenty of barbershops around where you can have a decent shave (although most barbers will object to the cigar thing).

WANTING TO HELP

Everywhere I look, I see men either crushed under a staggering amount of work or rejecting responsibility and doing appalling damage to their loved ones.

I'm not foolish enough to think I have the answer to this. But I know that miserable men spread misery around them, so maybe one answer could be to make men happier.

So the question becomes: how do you make men happier?

There's no single answer to this either, and probably most of it lies on a spiritual plane (contrary to popular belief, you cannot make yourself happy with a Lamborghini). But if you are interested in the physical side of life, consider this. The single most frequently used tool for men on this planet is the razor. It's sharp and can be dangerous. It can inspire fear, lack of confidence and general ill-humour. And you're expected to use one before breakfast. Most importantly, it's the only tool I really know how to handle, so the only way I can help the lumbering mass of Western men is to give them some tips on shaving.

Then think of this: if you pick up even one tip from this book, you'll benefit from it nearly every day of your life. I think that's worthwhile – it's what kept me going sometimes at four in the morning.

And that's all I've got. Farewell and shave well.

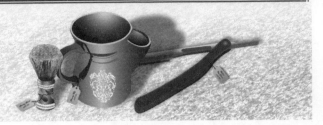

I've decided to include a list of shops where you can purchase some or all of the products mentioned in this book. Some have physical locations, but I recommend sourcing most on the web. I find it's easier and you have a wider selection than if you limit yourself to one shop. Happy hunting.

The Gentleman's Shop

Charnham House, 29–30 Charnham Street, Hungerford
Berkshire RG17 0EJ
www.gentlemans-shop.com
All shaving products.

Taylor of Old Bond Street

74 Jermyn Street, London SW1Y 6NP
www.tayloroldbondst.co.uk
All shaving products.

GEO. F. TRUMPER

9 Curzon Street, London W1J 5HQ, and

Geo. F. Trumper, 20 Jermyn Street, London SW1Y 6HP

www.trumpers.com

All shaving products.

PAUL MOLÉ

1031 Lexington Avenue

New York

NY 10021

For a classic, luxurious shave.

L'OCCITANE

Multiple locations globally

www.loccitane.com

Good for shaving cream and

aftershaves. Also sell styptic sticks.

THE ART OF SHAVING

373 Madison Avenue, New York, NY 10017

www.theartofshaving.com

All shaving products.

www.amazingshaving.com

Online shop selling all shaving products.

www.classicshaving.com

Online shop selling all shaving products.

www.shavemac.com

Online shop selling all shaving products.

Books Referred To

Iron John: Men and Masculinity
Bly, Robert
Sydney, Addison-Wesley Publishing Company Inc. 1990,
ISBN 0-7126-1070-7

On Becoming a Person: A Therapist's View of Psychotherapy
Rogers, Carl R.
London, Constable & Co. 1961, ISBN 0094604401

A Book of Five Rings
Musashi, Miyamoto
New York, Shambhala Publications Inc, 1994, ISBN 0877739986

God and the State
Bakunin, Michael
London, Dover Publications, 1970, ISBN 048622483X

The Razor Edge Book of Sharpening
Juranitch, John
New York, Warner Books Inc, 1985, ISBN 0-446-38002-4 (USA)
0-446-38003-2 (Canada)